P9-DHA-763

Integrated Chiropractic Technique: Chiropraxis

Predecessor text: *Chiropraxis, 1994;* revised 2001, 2005, 2009
Reprinting 2012

Address correspondence to:
Robert Cooperstein, M.A., D.C.
Palmer College of Chiropractic West Campus
90 East Tasman Avenue
San Jose CA 95134

on the web: chiropraxis.com
e-mail cooperstein_r@palmer.edu

Integrated Chiropractic Technique: Chiropraxis

The term *Chiropraxis* refers to an integrated practice of chiropractic theory and theory of chiropractic practice. Chiropraxis attempts to tie together much of what has been assimilated in a rather disconnected manner into a general model that leaves behind the pitfalls of the "brand-name" techniques - the infantile claims for uniqueness, originality, superiority, etc.

My most focused effort has been an attempt to describe how the body enters into coherent distortion patterns given some disruption of its postural homeostasis. This project has been a response to an unfortunate tendency for many chiropractors and chiropractic students to regard the body as a pile of bones that either stack up properly or don't, as if each bone had an independent say as to where it ought to be.

The first edition of *Chiropraxis* was published in 1990, and received major revisions in 2000 and again in 2004, when I changed the text enough to warrant a new title: *Integrated Chiropractic Technique: Chiropraxis.* The current revision incorporates material from several articles that I published in various places, has some new writing (for example, a new chapter on the temporomandibular joint), and considerable rearranging of older material to make for a better flow.

I would like to thank a few people for their help, rendered in various ways. Michael Hickey, John Badanes, Elaine Cooperstein, and countless chiropractic students and chiropractors whom I have met and with whom I have had correspondence along the way.

> *"Why are these people laughing?"*
> Dr. D.H. Badanes
> (The Evil One)

Integrated Chiropractic Technique: Chiropraxis

TABLE OF CONTENTS

1. Integrated Chiropractic Technique

It is commonly stated that chiropractic is an art, science, and philosophy. Chiropractic technique can be understood as the integration of all three components: the thoughtful application of scientific understanding to chiropractic patient care. It combines the practice of chiropractic theory and the theory of chiropractic practice. In the century plus that chiropractic has been around, it is no exaggeration to state that hundreds of different named technique systems have been devised: the Gonstead Technique, the Palmer Method, Sacro-Occipital Technique, and so on. Most of these brand-name (or proprietary) techniques claim to be superior to the others, and to treat a great variety of (if not all) health problems without needing treatment methods that would be found in a different technique system.

On the other hand, in the absence of any evidence that any one technique system is superior to any other, at least for all patients in all possible clinical situations, many chiropractors have become very comfortable mixing and combining technique procedures (both evaluative and adjustive) from among the many technique systems. This type of rational eclecticism is central to modern chiropractic technique, and we have come to call this technique Integrated Chiropractic Technique, or ICT for short.

ICT is eclectic and systematic

It is commonly stated that since no one technique will work for all doctors, nor get good results with all patients, that every doctor should learn at least "a couple" of techniques. We wholeheartedly agree, and go one step further: we feel a successful doctor should be able to draw from many, many

> Integrated Chiropractic Technique
> * A diversified, meaning eclectic approach
> * Synthesizes technique procedures from many technique systems
> * Integrates technique procedures and world views
> * Analytic and adjustive cornerstones

techniques, where each chiropractic adjustive procedure is made richer through integration with others. We like to think of this process as cross-fertilization, and the resultant technique hybrid vigor is what explains the success of our technique program.

The public is often confused by the great variety of chiropractic techniques, which no doubt dissuades some from seeking chiropractic care. Medical doctors, for similar reasons, are sometimes reluctant to refer patients to chiropractors. Health insurers increasingly expect of the chiropractic profession a more standardized approach to administering health care. We are fully aware of these situations, and how they are likely to affect the professional success of our chiropractic graduates. Therefore, we strive with great diligence to ensure that the chiropractic technique we teach is safe, effective, scientifically defensible, and widely practiced. We want our graduates not only well trained in the mainstream chiropractic techniques, but prepared to administer them in a contemporary health care setting that more and more emphasizes a rational integration of traditional chiropractic methods into a versatile and diverse armamentarium.

Although no one technique system can do it all, that does not mean chiropractic technique should be anything less than systematic. We believe it is possible to approach patients with a systematic method that is also eclectic. Clinical protocols can and have been devised for managing patients with various presenting signs and symptoms; i.e., conditions. Furthermore, there are certain diagnostic/analytic and adjustive cornerstones that would mostly be implemented in a similar manner irrespective of particular conditions, that may be termed subluxation-based care. Indeed, these pages are largely confined to just these practically universal cornerstones, since condition-based care must be addressed in a clinic setting, not a technique class.

Why "ICT" ?

When asked what chiropractic technique I prefer, I wish I could simply answer "Diversified." That would convey the sense of "eclectic," meaning I use bits and pieces of everything I have ever learned by studying and using a great variety of chiropractic techniques, both named Techniques (upper case T) and generic technique procedures (lower case t). Unfortunately, as appealing as this would be, it might lead to some misunderstanding. This would be due to the fact that Diversified technique has led a dual existence almost from the beginning. It can be seen as a standalone technique, parallel to other technique systems, such as Gonstead or Activator; or it can be be considered an umbrella for virtually all things chiropractic. I have written about this duality a few times, most specifically in a journal article (1).

At some point I began stated I used integrated methods, or practiced "Integrated Technique." It conveys the same sense as "Diversified" as an umbrella term. That best describes what I do: a little bit of this, and a little bit of that. I hope that is clear.

ICT analytic and adjustive cornerstones

ICT has certain cornerstones, in terms of both analysis and treatment procedures. I cover these in chapters 2 and 3 respectively. The analytic cornerstones have been summarized in the PARTS acronym (2), which has become very popular in chiropractic technique and has also been endorsed by Medicare. Osteopathy has developed a similar conceptual tool, and calls it the TART acronym. The procedural cornerstones amount to a series considerations and often competing paradigms on how best to treat patients.

Analytic cornerstones (chapter 2)

postural evaluation
global range of motion
pain and tenderness
segmental findings
segmental palpatory findings (misalignment and fixation)
ortho-neurological findings
interpretation of pain-provocation patterns
radiographic findings
reflex findings
identification of kinetic chains

Adjustive cornerstones (chapter 3)

manipulation / adjustment as appropriate
leverage
patient selection
doctor selection
assisted and resisted adjustments
joint kinematics (synkinetic adjusting)
structural findings
segmental intervention
regional intervention
rehabilitative procedures
case management
addressing kinetic chains

Subluxation

Much blood has been spilled among chiropractors on just what it is they treat, or even if they "treat." Some would say that they address a variety of conditions, not unlike those addressed by allopathic professions, although the treatment methods are different. Others would say that chiropractic, by definition, addresses subluxation, the root cause of the conditions in question. ICT believes the following definition of subluxation, the outcome of consensus proceedings facilitated by Dr. Meridel Gatterman, serves the needs of this text well:

Subluxation is:

1. Partial or incomplete dislocation.
2. Restriction of motion of a joint in a position exceeding normal physiologic motion, although the anatomic limits have not been exceeded.
3. Aberrant relationship between two adjacent articular structures, which may have functional or pathological sequella, causing an alternation in the biomechanical and/or neurophysiological reflexes of these articular structures, their proximal structures, and/or body systems that may be directly or indirectly affected by them.

The Association of Chiropractic Colleges also provides a definition which by definition suits virtually all the North American chiropractic colleges. The ACC's has adopted the following paradigm statements regarding subluxation:

> Chiropractic is Concerned with the preservation and restoration of health, and focuses particular attention on the subluxation.

> A subluxation is a complex of functional and/or structural and/or pathological articular changes that compromise neural integrity and may influence organ system function and general health.

> A subluxation is evaluated, diagnosed, and managed through the use of chiropractic procedures based on the best available rational and empirical evidence.

Listings

In common parlance a "listing" is a direction of tilt, a leaning to one side. Chiropractors have been using this word since the beginning to describe the direction in which a vertebra has misaligned with respect to...with respect to - something! Obviously, a segment can be misaligned only with respect to some other reference point: the segment above or below, the floor, perhaps the central ray of the x-ray tube. It would be an understatement to say that chiropractors have not always been able to agree upon a standard listings system; on the contrary, a rather byzantine discussion over many years has led to very little.

Several factors have interacted to confuse the discussion:

• as mentioned above, there has been a lack of a common reference point for listings;

• there are many different methods for obtaining listings (x-ray, motion palpation, static palpation, muscle palpation, reflex methods employing leg checks, challenges;

• some practitioners use the vertebral body and others use the vertebral spinous process as the reference point for their nomenclatural system.

Nomenclatural Rules or Kinematics?

Certain nomenclatural rules have been adopted merely in order that discussion of mechanical matters may begin. For example, let us suppose that a segment can be seen on a spinograph to reside anteriorward in relationship to the segment below. Should I describe this situation in terms of an anteriority of the superior segment, or a posteriority of the inferior segment? It has become established, among medical doctors as well as chiropractors, that this should be termed an anterolisthesis of the segment above. Unfortunately, this merely nomenclatural rule is seen by many to contain mechanical significance, generally that it is the superior segment which has subluxated, and should be contacted in the event of a corrective thrust.

The terminological convention should not imply that the underlying biomechanical fault resides in the one segment rather than the other, insofar as the subluxation occurs in the joint between the two. Furthermore, there is no a priori reason to suppose that when a clinician attempts to reduce the subluxation by applying a thrust that the force which is applied moves a segment with respect to the one below, any more than with respect to the segment above. Cineradiography has demonstrated that a manipulative thrust introduces a damped disturbance into the spine which extends to several motor units both above and below the point of contact, although it affects the immediately adjacent articulations the most. It's one thing to list L4 with respect to L5, but quite another to suppose that a contact on L4 affects primarily the joint between the two (as opposed to L3-4).
In addressing the analytic and adjustive principles with which we deal on a daily

basis, nothing is more central than the concept of listings. These amount to indications for adjustive care.

Static

In the language of daily life, a "listing" is a direction of tilt, a leaning to one side of the vertebrae. One presumes that the chiropractic started out just this way, although at this time the term listing is also used to describe rotational misalignments and even joint fixations, which need not be about vertebral positions at all! Chiropractors use the word "listing" to describe the direction in which a vertebra has misaligned with respect to...with respect to - something! Obviously, a segment can be misaligned only with respect to some other reference point: the segment above or below, the floor, perhaps the central ray of the x-ray tube. It would be an understatement to say that chiropractors have often disagreed on how to create a standard listings system. Nevertheless, among the several systems that have been created, ICT emphasizes the Gonstead-Palmer system for static listings (misalignment) and the language of restrictions for dynamic findings, as used in motion palpation. It is important to note that in both static and dynamic listings systems, as a convention, we list the bone above in relation to the one below. That doesn't mean the upper bone is the "subluxated" or "dysfunctional" vertebra; rather, that the we have all agreed to describe the problem with the articulation from the vantage point of the superior segment. Medical radiologists have adopted the same convention.

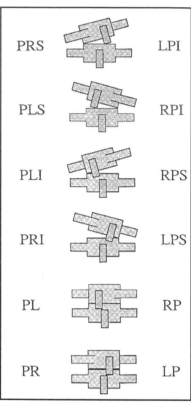

Palmer-Gonstead (left) and National (right) static listings system, C2-L5

The figure to the right depicts the Palmer-Gonstead and National listings for C2-L5. The great majority of chiropractors are likely to be comfortable with these, judging from the finding of the National Board of Chiropractic Examiners' finding that "Diversified" is the most practiced of chiropractic techniques (91% of respondents to a survey said they had used it within the last 2 years).

Remember: these are static listings, dynamic listings are described below.

Three letter" and "four letter" listings systems are usually used for the atlanto-occipital and C1-2 listings, respectively, not herein described; likewise, there are sacral and sacroiliac listings as well, also not described (obviously there is much work to do!). Many technique systems employ their own distinct terminology (SOT, CBP, Thompson, Activator, etc.) but it is beyond our scope to go into these at this time. We return to this in a later chapter.

Dynamic (motion palpation listings)

Several systems have been developed that have in common the fact that it is the function of the motor unit, rather than the position of any particular bone, that forms the reference point for the listing. With respect to the segment below, a segment is listed as hypomobile or hypermobile in one or more of the six degrees of freedom that are theoretically possible. There are three possibilities for linear translation and three axes around which rotation make take place. In practice, the rotations are stressed, such that a segment is generally listed as exhibiting improper motion in either lateral flexion. forward flexion, extension, or rotation about the vertical (y) axis or combination thereof. The diagram below depicts these relationships.

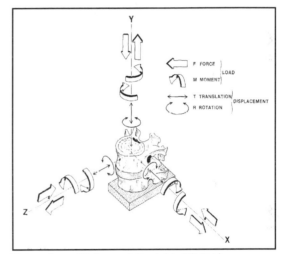

Taken from White and Panjabi. *Clinical Biomechanics of the Spine*

The word restriction is central to our understanding of this system: a vertebral segment is defined as restricted in the direction it will not adequately move. For example, a vertebra that does not engage in normal left lateral flexion is restricted in "left lateral flexion." The only reason one needs to make this rather obvious point is that there is occasionally confusion on this point, with some erroneously believing that restriction on the left would prevent bending to the right. (Remember, the point in this last sentence is incorrect!)

Sticky joints or crooked bones?

Although throughout most of its history chiropractic emphasized vertebral misalignment as the primary pathology addressed, there has been something of a paradigm shift in the last two decades in which many have come to the conclusion that intervertebral joint function (especially fixation, or loss of movement capacity) may be of greater significance. No doubt the two are intimately related, so that vertebral misalignment could result in impaired movement, while impaired movement in turn could lead to misalignment. However there is no reason to insist that both must be present in every situation. It is very likely that a given spinal unit in a given patient may be misaligned but fully mobile, while another may be hypomobile but in perfect alignment, while another may be misaligned and hypomobile. In any case, in spite of much speculation and unrestrained assuming, no one has been able to discover or produce a chiropractic "Rosetta stone" that would allow us to predict specific misalignments from identified fixations, or predict specific directions of fixation from identified misalignments. ICT aims at identifying "sticky joints" and "crooked bones" (as Dr. Stonebrink, retired technique maven at Western States Chiropractic College, once put it), and resists the temptation to rely on simplistic rules that purport to relate the one type of finding to the other.

Some clinicians assess the movement properties of the spine less to identify fixations per se, and more to infer static misalignment from these dynamic faults. In other words, their primary purpose is not to identify fixations as adjustable entities, but rather to predict specific misalignments from specific fixations. Even though the examination procedure involves motion assessment, the goal of the adjustment is not so much to restore movement as to realign the spine. ICT believes such procedures to be very error prone, and adopts the straightforward position – at least until the dynamic-to-static Rosetta stone is revealed – that fixation is a stand alone entity, to be treated as such, and likewise for misalignment. So: for us, as an example, the detection of reduced lateral flexion does not imply an ipsilateral "open wedge," nor does impaired rotation in a given direction predict a "PR" or a "PL." All such rules, no matter how traditional, remain hypotheses at the current time.

Segmentalism or structuralism?

Again, throughout most of its history, starting with the Palmers, chiropractic has emphasized segmental subluxations (however that term be defined), spinal problems attributed to two adjacent vertebra and the related soft tissues. (Of course, this was generalized to include the atlanto-occipital, lumbosacral, and sacroiliac joints as well, and quite often to the extremity joints.) On the other hand, there always was a structuralist tendency as well, probably starting with the work of Dr. Willard Carver, that emphasized spinal regional considerations, and beyond that, the relation of the various spinal regions to one another.

The segmentalist believes that cranial-spinal-pelvic subluxations occur at specific motor units consisting of two bones, be they vertebrae, the skull, any of the pelvic bones, or combinations thereof. As a general rule, the segment above is characterized with respect to the one below, whether simply in order to generate a determinate but pathomechanically neutral language of listings, or whether out of some pathomechanical conception governing the nature of the misalignment. The subluxation in the specific motor unit results in postural distortions such as scoliosis in the frontal plane, and loss or exaggeration of the two kyphotic and two lordotic curves in the sagittal plane. These postural distortions are seen as compensatory consequences of specific motor unit subluxations, and not as the problems in and of themselves. Gonstead is the classic example.

The posturalist precisely sees postural distortion as the subluxation in and of itself, and offers up a language of listings which describes the linear and angular relationship of entire regions of the cranial-spinal-pelvic articulations. A given motor unit may exhibit more signs and symptoms of dysfunction than another, but this is the consequence rather than the cause of the primary postural distortion. For example, the apex of a lateral curvature in the frontal plane may present with more pain, and show more osteophytosis on an x-ray, than the other segments which comprise the curvature. Nonetheless, the curvature, and not its apex, is the subluxation. The posturalist claims that the spine subluxates as groupings of adjacent vertebrae, and is to be adjusted accordingly, with relatively non-specific contacts. Pettibon's Spinal Biomechanics technique is the classic example.

ICT does not feel the need to choose between segmentalist and structuralist thinking, to wind up at either of these two extreme positions. It is more likely that given patients are better understood as suffering from either segmental or regional complaints; that a segmental problem is very much affected by the local environment in which it occurs, just as the local spinal environment is partially governed by segmental problems. The table below illustrates how the segmentalist/structuralist dimension intersects the misalignment/fixation dimension, and gives examples of descriptive listings.

	segmentalist approach	**structuralist approach**
alignment problem	L3-4 misalignment	lumbar curvature (scoliosis)
movement problem	L3-4 fixation	unilateral reduced lumbar lateral flexion

Segmental evaluation

There are many dimensions in which spinal segments may be assessed: static position, dynamic movement, soft tissue texture and quality, visualization, pain and tenderness, etc. Although we cannot go into the intricacies of these assessment procedures here and now, it must be noted that most of the studies addressing the interexaminer reliability of segmental findings, with the exception of pain and tenderness, have *not* found them very reproducible. It seems that the broader the question, the more easily the parameter can be measured and the more likely the examiners to agree: global range of motion, postural evaluation, etc. (discussed below). Nonetheless, there will always be a place for segmental evaluation, the difficulties notwithstanding, if for no other reason than that some patients suffer from problems that are best understood as segmental (at least in this author's opinion).

The primary two segmental findings have to with position and movement (we have already warned against trying to derive one from the other). One would think that the gold standard evaluation for position would be x-ray, certainly as compared with manual palpation, but even that is controversial. People have questioned the reproducibility of patient positioning, the interexaminer reliability of x-ray interpretation (i.e., line marking), the validity of radiographic findings as it relates to patients, and finally, the clinical utility of x-ray (is the outcome of patient care ultimately made better by the use of x-rays?). Since in any case, x-rays can not be taken on every office visit, one presumes chiropractors will continue to use manual palpation to determine vertebral positions.

As for motion palpation for segmental hyper- or hypomobility, again, there have been substantial interexaminer reliability problems, a fact unnecessary to belabor. On the other hand, given the primacy of segmental motion palpation in the core curricula of most of the chiropractic colleges, and its continued heavy usage among field doctors, it displays no tendency to become any less important. Moreover, the central thesis of segmental motion palpation, that it ought to be possible to manually assess the quantity and quality of joint movement, is so inherently plausible that it is probably worth the effort to evaluate and improve this examination method. Some examiners concentrate on joint excursion, the magnitude of linear and angular movements in all the relevant directions. Others are more concerned with the quality of joint motions, especially end-feel (hard or soft), and accessory joint movements (into the paraphysiological joint space). Paradoxically, it appears that an intervertebral joint that has an abnormally hard end-feel may exhibit more excursion than its equal but opposite partner on the other side of the body.

Yes we know, thou shalt not adjust a hypermobile segment. Nevertheless, there are a few considerations to take into account. First, we can't justify taking stress x-rays, the gold standard for identifying instability, on every patient. Second, it is at best hard to palpate for hypermobility. That stated, even with reasonable certainty that there is instability, it may not be present in all the degrees of freedom for the joint in question. For example, T8-9 may be hypermobile in left lateral flexion, yet hypomobile in right lateral flexion. Many think such relationships are virtually the rule, rather than a surprising finding. Therefore, perhaps the commandment above should be restated as "Thou shalt not adjust a hypermobile joint in a direction that puts further stress on its restraining soft tissues, although other lines of drive may be indicated."

The other commandment, to the effect that thou shalt adjust only fixations, is probably less controversial. One would, of course, take into account that some patients have congenital or acquired ankylosis, age-related and other contraindications, histories of surgery, etc. When all is said and done, it is likely better that joints be mobile than restricted, and there are good laboratory data showing that laboratory-fixed joints begin to degenerate almost immediately. We must note, however, that sometimes instability results in splinting spasm that an examiner would detect as "restriction," and when that is the case (and no one says this will be a simple clinical scenario to unravel!), the *initial* goal of care may be related to soft-tissue intervention.

Postural evaluation

Postural faults result in abnormal stresses on soft tissues and joints by maintaining them in non-neutral positions for potentially long periods of time. In the frontal plane, this often results in spinal curvature (scoliosis) and lateral inclination; in the sagittal plane, this results in exaggerated or diminished kyphotic and lordotic curves. Manipulative thrusts should be delivered so as to diminish the stretch on abnormally elongated tissues, and so as to stretch contractured tissue.

Congruency of examination findings

Ideally, all the different examination findings would provide congruent information, would tell the same story. In the real world, incongruency is a way of life, which means the doctor must be emotionally and intellectually prepared to make decisions based on imperfect information. Better that, than reinterpret the data or redo examination procedures in a futile attempt to make things fit. We tend to have some hierarchy in our minds as to the relative importance of the different types of diagnostic procedures. No doubt there is room for significant differences among doctors, whereby one may emphasize orthopedic information over segmental evaluation, and the other vice versa. Someday, based on improvements in examination techniques, especially in objective measurements, it may be possible to identify which types of findings are the most predictive of the others, and thus the most clinically useful. Until then, we will just have to make do with what we have, our examination methods as they are and our capacity to live with some degree of uncertainty.

Specificity

Much blood has been spilt in chiropractic on the notion of specificity. The concept of specificity has been central to chiropractic technique since the time of D.D. Palmer. To this day, the technique rooms at Palmer Davenport have

Specificity
•   Adjustive: where is the segmental contact, what moves?
•   Diagnostic: what level or region is implicated by an exam procedure?
•   A matter of consistency between test and adjustive procedure

feature placards advising "Chiropractic is specific or it is nothing," attributed to B.J. Palmer, in his Volume XVIII of the green book series.

Specificity can be viewed in a number of ways. Adjustive specificity has to do with our ability to deliver a force to an intended spinal target, without inadvertently affecting areas of the spine, at least not very much. It also refers to the intention to deploy a given vector, a controlled force with an intentional direction and amplitude. It is not well-established that safe and effective clinical outcomes depend on a high level of adjustive specificity, despite our historical adherence to this concept. Diagnostic specificity has to do with our ability to reliably implicate the same spinal segment or articulation during examination procedures. Again, It is not well-established that safe and effective clinical outcomes depend on a high level of diagnostic specificity. Indeed, it is difficult to explain the apparent success of a great variety of chiropractic adjustive procedures, when demonstrated low levels of interexaminer reliability in widely used examination procedures suggests the notion of a specific chiropractic diagnosis (i.e., "listing") may be more wishful thinking than reality.

As research continues in the area of diagnostic and adjustive specificities, let us point out that the concept of specificity is not synonymous with that of segmentalism. The great structuralist chiropractic Mortimer Levine Levine hated being accused of practicing "general adjusting," as distinguished from the vaunted "specific adjusting. He said that he was being just as specific in his postural approach as chiropractors using a segmental approach. "As long as an adjusting [sic] is applied according to a corrective hypothesis after analysis of the patient's distortion, that adjusting is specific" (3) (p. 88). For Levine, general adjusting meant using a postural approach to chiropractic, nothing more, nothing less. It was to be judged not according to some petrified, pseudo-philosophical definition of segmental specificity, but on its own merits, according to how its use affected clinical outcomes.

Listings systems used by chiropractic techniques

Because of the complexities involved, only the main determinants of a few of the main systems can herein be described. It should be noted that each has various exceptions and "special listings" that embrace specific segments and particular unusual mechanical events. In some ways it turns out that frequently, but certainly not always, discussing listings is tantamount to discussing chiropractic spinography, insofar as many listings are automatically generated by the x-ray line marking analyses peculiar to the given technique. It also turns out that so much of a given technique's mechanical theory - or perhaps lack thereof - is bound up in its listing system, that no critical look may be afforded the latter without simultaneously critiquing the mechanical conceptions themselves. The reader is asked to tolerate the extent to which a mere review of listings devolves into a critical analysis of spinographic technique and mechanical conceptions.

Gonstead

Two points need to be made immediately. First, the Gonstead system posits a certain mechanical assumption (of questionable validity) that underlies everything: a vertebra, in the process of subluxating, first "goes posterior," then possibly "rotates" and finally perhaps "wedges"; this means that all vertebral listings will include a vector of posteriority. Second, the spinous process rather than the body of the vertebra forms the anatomical frame of reference.

Thus, each vertebra (except C1) has a "three letter listing," the first of which is P for posterior, the second of which is either R or L to indicate whether the spinous process has rotated to the left or the right, and the third of which is either S or I to indicate whether the disc plane lines converge or diverge on the side of spinous rotation. For instance, the typical listing "PRS L2" signifies that the second lumbar has subluxated posteriorly with respect to L3, and has rotated and laterally flexed its body to the left.

It should be noted that this posteriority need not be observed on the lateral view. Likewise, the possibility of anterior subluxation is more or less dismissed, despite the following facts:

• Vertebra typically glide anterior in forward flexion, and in fact may become fixed in such a state of anterolisthetic flexion;

• Spinographic studies not uncommonly exhibit evidence of spondylolisthesis, both spondylolytic and non-spondylolytic.

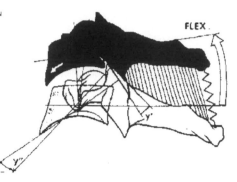

We see in Kapandji's drawing, that forward flexion in the neck is accompanied by anterior glide, creating the possibility of subluxations in which the superior segment is anterior.

In other words, anterior translation is one of the six degrees of freedom available to a vertebral segment; given that a broad consensus of chiropractors would agree that fixation subluxations occur when a segment "freezes" within the range of normal physiological motion, there are a priori reasons to object to the stipulation that posteriority is the rule.

Since the vertebra are constrained to subluxate posteriorly with respect to the segment below, and are barred from subluxating anteriorly, one is at a loss to explain how it is that L5 is permitted to subluxate anteriorly with respect to the sacral base. This lack of parallelism is all the more surprising since the lumbosacral joint is quite homologous to the intervertebral joints in general.

Let us note that the spinous process listings are determined purely in relationship to the central ray of the x-ray tube, so that a given segment that is not rotated with respect to the segment above or below will nonetheless be assigned a rotational malposition listing merely because it happens to be laterally tipped "off the level base." In other words, once it has been determined that a segment must indeed be listed - whether because the spinograph shows it has "wedged," or perhaps because there are clinical findings (instrumentation, palpation, etc.), its rotation is assessed by noting the location of the spinous process relative to the pedicles and the width of the vertebra considered in isolation from adjacent vertebrae.

The innominate bones are listed first as having gone either posteroinferior or anterosuperior, and then "internal" or "external" (medial or lateral) at the sacroiliac joint. The anatomical unlikelihood of a posteriorinferolateral subluxation or an anterosuperomedial subluxation is not considered, in spite of the fact that the sacroiliac joints converge posteriorly rather than align parallel to the sagittal plane.

The sacrum is listed with respect to the sacroiliac articulations or the lumbosacral joint. In the case of the "posterior sacrum," there is no mutual opposed innominate rotation, but the sacrum is said to have rotated posteriorly in the plane of its base on one side: in a P-L sacrum, the sacral base is posterior on the left, and the sacral tubercles are rotated to the right. After having rotated posteriorly, the sacral base may subluxate inferiorly as well, giving rise to the listing PI-L, meaning the sacrum is posterior and inferior on the left. No consideration is given to the possibility of an anterior sacrum (as described by Logan), and no consideration is given to the anatomical limitation that the sacral base, which is wider anteriorly than posteriorly, would force the ilia apart by a wedge action were it to subluxate posteriorly, an occurrence that would be strongly opposed by the powerful sacroiliac ligament.

The sacral listing with respect to the fifth lumbar vertebra is a "posterior sacral base," or "base posterior." Herbst (Sacral Misalignments, p.46) distinguishes a posterior sacral base from a spondylolytic spondylolisthesis of L5 in language that suggests that the Gonstead base posterior is in fact a nonspondylolytic spondylolisthesis. No consideration is given to the possibility of an anteriority of the sacral base with respect to the innominate bone.

The atlas listings are essentially identical to the listing system developed by toggle practitioners, and is described below in the section devoted to them. However, an important distinction in the interpretation of the listing needs to be made: the Gonstead listing is of atlas with respect to axis, whereas the upper cervical practitioners are listing atlas with respect to the occiput. Herbst writes: "A prevalent belief among many chiropractors is that when the atlas becomes subluxated it does so by slipping out from under, and thereby misaligning with, the occiput... [whereas in reality] an atlas subluxation occurs from the atlas misaligning with the axis."[1] The occiput, more or less like a vertebra, is said to wedge and rotate with respect to atlas, after having flexed anteriorly or extended.

Before leaving this description of Gonstead listings, we should mention that it is in very common use, not only among Gonstead clinicians but among Diversified and many other practitioners as well. As has been briefly mentioned above, certain anatomic, referential, and terminological ambiguities and uncertainties exist within it that wind up contradicting important tenets of other listing systems, including that of Logan and of Thompson. In the next unit we offer up a reconciliatory model, one which departs from certain conventional belief systems concerning the interpretation of the various listing systems, but which more than makes up for the departure by uniting them mechanically.

---

[1]Herbst A. Gonstead chiropractic science and art: the chiropractic methodology of Clarence S. Gonstead. Mount Horeb WI: Schichi Publications; 1980, p. 115-116.

Toggle/Upper Cervical

Atlas listings are derived from an analytic x-ray series: an upper cervical specific series, consisting of a lateral cervical, a vertex, and a nasium view. The nasium view is taken with caudad tube tilt, at an angle conforming to the plane line of atlas that is visualized in the lateral view. The vertex view is taken with the central ray more or less perpendicular to the surface of atlas.

Atlas listings consist of four letters. The first letter is always A, to indicate that when atlas subluxates it always glides anterior with respect to the occipital condyles. The second letter is either S or I, depending on whether the lateral view atlas plane line has tilted superior or inferior with respect to some norm (what norm?). The third letter is either L or R, depending on whether the nasium view shows the atlas to have translated either right or left with respect to the occipital condyles. The fourth and final letter is either P or A, denoting whether the atlas transverse process has rotated anteriorly or posteriorly on the side of laterality, as seen on the vertex view; this information is derived either from a vertex view or from the nasium, where it may be deduced based on the relative widths of the lateral masses (the wider lateral mass is said to be anterior).

Logan Technique[2]

In the end the Logan practitioner is going to list and quantify the degree of sacral inferiority, taking into account other mechanical complications such as "true pelvic anteriority." Neo-Logan practitioners, like Gonstead, have developed a full spine method of analyzing spinographs. Given that Logan mechanotherapeutics are almost entirely devoted to normalizing the inferiority of the sacrum (using the "Basic Contact" on the sacral apex and possibly a heel or sole lift to normalize the inferior sacrum) not surprisingly the spinographic analysis and the listings that are generated by it greatly emphasize the lumbopelvic area. The x-ray marking system is considerably more subtle than the Gonstead system which developed out of it, in that Logan has internal rules for detecting and "correcting" x-ray distortional effects that arise from the subject being off-center with respect to the central ray of the x-ray tube. Gonstead has borrowed correctional rules for pelvic torsional effects on femur head height (whether these rules are right or wrong) but not for left/right off centering.

In terms of listings, we need only mention that the determination of vertebral rotation depends on the location of the spinous process not with respect to the

---

[2]Filson RM, Johnson G. Technique system overview: Logan system of body mechanics assessment. Chiropractic Technique 1994;6(3):98-103.

central ray, as in Gonstead, but with respect to the location of the spinous processes above and below. Barge uses the same system throughout the spine, measuring the distance between the lateral aspect of the vertebra and the spinous process, comparing the left/right measurements for analogous measurements above and below. (See any of Dr. Barge's three related books, *Torticollis, Tortipelvis* or Scoliosis.)

Diversified

There isn t really a definite constituted Diversified listings system, anymore than there is a clearly defined Diversified technique per se. More often than not these practitioners employ Gonstead listings, using the spinous processes as reference points, with the main exception occurring in the neck where malpositions are designated with respect to the vertebral bodies. The vertebra are listed as "body right" or "body left" with respect to the segment below. A typical listing might be 'RPI" - body posterior on the right, closed wedge. As compared with Gonstead listings less information is conveyed, insofar as no information is presented concerning lateral curvatures ("wedging") should there be any present. The Gonstead doctor employs a line of drive that is toward the convexity of the spine, using a segmental contact point that takes the rotatory component into account, whereas the Diversified doctor simply adjusts (at least in the neck) according to the direction of vertebral rotation, not taking wedging into account. (We will explore the mechanical consequences of this methodology in the unit concerned with the cervical spine.)

Diversified practitioners, in addition to borrowing Gonstead listings, quite commonly make use of Derifield listings that are often imported from the context of the Thompson technique. (These latter will be examined below, in the unit devoted to the Derifield leg check and Thompsonian derivations.) There is a certain logic to this, insofar as Thompson and allied drop-table practitioners are phylogenetically within the Diversified camp. The use of the table does not itself alter the fundamental chiropractic world view of the practitioners: segments misalign, possibly resulting in nerve interference; the doctor adjusts the segment back toward "correction." Little if any attention is devoted to posture, and even less to the pathophysiology of the subluxation or kinetics of the correction (apart from the empty vague assertion that 'the table does the work." In other words, there is no constituted Diversified theory in the same sense for instance that there is a Logan, Gonstead, or Biomechanics theory.

Thompson Technique[3]

3

Pelvic syndrome is said to exist when the physiological short leg seems to lengthen with respect to the other when the patient s legs are flexed to approximately 90 degrees in the prone position. Cervical syndrome is said to exist when turning the prone patient s head to either the right or the left changes the apparent length of the legs. The syndrome is named according to which direction of rotation evens the apparent leg length, so that "right cervical syndrome" exists when turning the head to the right evens a short right or left leg. The doctor will locate a "painful nodule (or "taut and tender fibers") on the exposed side of the neck. The doctor s adjustment is applied to the lamina of the involved vertebra, which is to say he adjusts the segment as a "body left/right" according to the Diversified system of nomenclature.

It has occasionally been suggested that whereas pelvic positive would signify a "PI" ilium, pelvic negative would signify an "AS" ilium. Thompson himself appears to believe the latter to denote some sort of PI ilium with "sacral involvement," or some entity involving primarily hamstring spasm. It is our opinion (developed in the unit concerned with the Derifield leg check and Thompsonism) that both pelvic negative and pelvic positive signify PI iliums of possibly different ilk - but are still both PI iliurns. We have a vested interest, now that we have greatly complicated the mechanical model of the PT ilium PDS, to cling to a few empirical "rules," where it appears that the old and new conceptions coincide. It would be nice if we could agree that a physiological short leg, *ceterus paribus*, almost always indicates a PI ilium.

Pierce-Stillwagon technique very much resembles the Thompson work. It adds to the Thompson listings repertoire the "Double AS" and "Double PI" listings. which should not be understood as double sacroiliac lesions, but rather as lumbopelvic. x-ray derived descriptions of the overall arrangement. Double AS patients are hyperlordotic in the lumbar spine, whereas Double P1 patients are hypolordotic. Pierce adds the C5 listing, and thus the C5 adjustment, to the blend. At the end of the chapter is a flow chart showing how a typical drop table practice processes its patients, mostly drawn from a Pierce-Stillwagon technique manual. The reader is also referred to my article on the Thompson Technique, published in the journal *Chiropractic Technique.*[4]

Motion Palpation

Several systems have been developed that have in common the fact that it is the

---

[4]Cooperstein R. Technique system overview: Thompson Technique. Chiropractic Technique 1995;7(2):60-63.

function of the motor unit, rather than the position of any particular bone, that forms the reference point for the listing. A segment is listed as hypomobile or hypermobile with respect to the segment below, in one or more of the available motions that are theoretically possible. There are three possibilities for linear translation and three axes around which rotation make take place.

It should be noted that the practitioners of this type of listings system tend not to be overly concerned with the static initial spatial relationships that typify a given motor unit when they evaluate motion. In other words, a given articulation may exhibit hyperextension (by some definition) in the "neutral" position, but what concerns the examiner is whether starting from this position a segment is able to flex and extend normally. A hyperextended motor unit which nonetheless can be assessed to maintain normal dynamic extensibility would be found normal in that regard, and it might turn out to be hypomobile in forward flexion (for example).

Houston Codes

This system of listings was originally developed by Howe and Hildebrandt to describe for the most part spinographic findings, although some of the categories refer to motor units that display aberrant motion. Although seemingly straight-forward, this listings system has been poorly received by many chiropractors who see it as somehow "pro-medical." (Representative quotation: "At this date 1197Os1 the Americans who had this method forced on them by Medicare, are finding it very hard to live with due to the previously mentioned difficulty in constantly proving the subluxation. May we in Canada never fall into this trap.[5] The listings in themselves are essentially self-explanatory and are as follows:

A. Static intersegmental subluxations
    1. Flexion malposition
    2. Extension malposition
    3. Lateral flexion malposition
    4. Rotational malposition
    5. Anterolisthesis
    6. Retrolisthesis
    7. Lateralisthesis
    8. Altered interosseous spacing (decreased/increased)
    9. Osseous foraminal encroachments

---

[5]MacRae JE. Roentgenometrics in Chiropractic. Toronto, Canada: Canadian Memorial Chiropractic College; 1974, p. 89.

B. Kinetic intersegmental subluxations
        1. Hypomobility (fixation subluxation)
        2. Hypermobility (loosened vertebral motor unit)
        3. Aberrant motion

C. Sectional subluxation
        1. Scoliosis and/or alterations of curves secondary to muscular imbalance
        2. Scoliosis and/or alterations of curves secondary to structural asymmetries
        3. Decompensation of adaptational curvatures
        4. Abnormalities of motion
D. Paravertebral subluxations
        1. Costovertebral and costotransverse disrelationships
        2. Sacroiliac subluxations

Right-handed Orthagonal (Cartesian) System

This system was proposed by White and Panjabi.[6] Chiropractors have by and large have found it too cumbersome to use, although Don Harrison (Biophysics technique) has endorsed it and the ACA Council on Technique has expressed serious interest in it. The typical clinician seems to feel that however useful this system is from a mathematical or biomechanical point of view, it does not improve upon traditional listing languages in a way that benefits field practitioners.

It is agreed as a convention that the coordinate system for describing the kinematics of the human spine is structured as follows: the origin is between the cornua of the sacrum. The x axis is horizontal and runs left/right, and is the axis about which forward flexion and extension takes place; the y axis is vertical and is the axis about which axial twisting takes place; and the z axis is, which is also horizontal, projects forward and back, and is the axis about which lateral bending takes place. The sagittal plane is determined by the z-y axes, the frontal plane by the x-y axes, and the transverse plane by the z-x axes. Movements that are forward along z, to the left along x, and up along y are defined as positive linear translations, and opposite directions of motion are defined as negative in value. Likewise, clockwise rotations about an axis are defined as + or - theta (theta is the angle of rotation), with the observer assumed to be standing at the origin looking in the direction of the positive direction of the axis. For example, + theta x corresponds to forward flexion, and right lateral flexion is + theta z.

---

[6]White AA, Panjabi MM. Clinical Biomechanics of the Spine. 1st ed. Philadelphia PA: J. B. Lippincott Company; 1978, p. 62-62.

Coupling is said to occur when a vertebra exhibits motion in more than one degree of freedom simultaneously, as when the cervical vertebrae translate anteriorly during flexion of the neck, forward (+ theta x coupled with +z). The fact that coupling occurs implies that the axis of rotation which may be described for a particular vertebral motion may itself be a function of time, in that its precise location changes during the time interval in which motion occurs.

Sacro-Occipital Technique

SOT is a vast technique, with lots of nooks and crannies. We do not dare get involved with nomenclature in the limited time and space available here, but we should mention the "category" system of patient classification. For a fuller description, with citations, see my article on SOT, published in the journal *Chiropractic Technique*.[7]

The category system serves as the lynch-pin of structural correction, while Chiropractic Manipulative Reflex Technique (CMRT) represents the mainstay of somatovisceral intervention. From a diagnostic point of view, the ascription of patients to one of three possible "categories" is central. Category I, "the first level of subluxation to develop" would involve failed coordination between the "sacroiliac respiratory motion" and the "cranial sacral respiratory mechanism," which are normally connected by virtue of the dural membranes and the flow of cerebral spinal fluid. Category II, following on the heels of an unresolved Category I subluxation, involves the "weight-bearing" function of the sacroiliac joint, and is essentially a post-traumatic clinical entity. It would "affect the connective tissue of the cranial sutures and spine, the iliofemoral ligaments, the extremities, and the psoas muscle." An unresolved Category II may progress to a Category III, characterized as an insult to the lumbosacral cartilaginous system, accompanied by

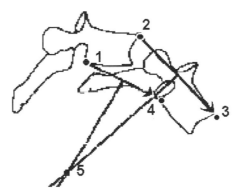

The IAR. Figure from White AA, Panjabi MM. Clinical Biomechanics of the Spine. 1st ed. Philadelphia PA: J. B. Lippincott Company; 1978.White and Pandjabi

nerve root compression or stretch syndrome, injury to "disc tissue, the surrounding muscles, the sciatic nerve and the pyriformis muscles." At the end of this chapter is a flow chart I prepared that shows the SOT category system of

---

[7]Cooperstein R. Technique system overview: Sacro Occipital Technique. Chiropractic Technique 1996;8(3):125-131.

patient classification. I apologize in advance for not being an expert in "boxology" as Dr. Dan Hansen puts it – on to *Visio!*

Instantaneous axis of rotation

The term instantaneous axis of rotation (IAR) has been defined to embrace this concept: this axis is perpendicular to the plane in which the rigid body moves. The perpendicular bisectors of any two lines connecting the original and new positions of any two points in the body determine this axis (again, see White and Panjabi). The location of this line and the angle describes the motion.

Notes

1.   Cooperstein R. Diversified technique: core of chiropractic or "just another technique system"? Journal of Chiropractic Humanities 1995;5(1):50-55.
2.   Bergmann T. P.A.R.T.S. joint assessment procedure. Chiropractic Technique 1993;5(3):135-136.
3.   Levine M. The Structural Approach to Chiropractic. New York, NY: The Comet Press, Inc.; 1964.

2. Analytic cornerstones

This chapter reviews the principal methods chiropractors use to evaluate the spine. A more detailed discussion can be found in (1), which has chapters on these principal methods: palpation, manual muscle testing, x-ray line marking, leg checking, thermography, and other forms of instrumentation.

The chiropractic analytic cornerstones have been summarized in the very popular PARTS acronym (2). Most of the procedures includes within PARTS can also be found in osteopathy and other forms of manual medicine. The procedures

```
PARTS
•      Pain
•      Asymmetry
•      Range of motion
•      Tone, Texture, Temperature change
•      Special tests
```

more unique to chiropractic tend to be covered under "special tests," and as has already been mentioned, are discussed in (1).

The art of spinal palpation

Most of the PARTS components are accessible using palpation. Spinal palpation is undertaken primarily to identify underlying segmental dysfunction. Abnormal autonomic reactions may permit the identification of involved areas with minimal palpatory pressure. An area which is painful to light \palpation, or which demonstrates erythema or increased sweating may be due to underlying spinal subluxation.

Objective palpation findings require a sound knowledge of the anatomical structures underlying the area being palpated. Palpatory pressure must also be modified depending upon the case, e.g., only light pressure should be used following an acute injury.

The requirements for accurate palpation should include the following:

• Any painful areas reported by the patient during the palpation procedure should be accurately localized and noted

• Any areas of swelling or edema should be carefully palpated and noted

- The skin over the spinal region should be palpated for any areas of increased temperature, indicating possible underlying segmental dysfunction or pathology;

- Muscles should be palpated for areas of hardness or palpable bands of fibrosis

- Static palpation of underlying osseous structures should be performed to identify alignment anomalies and areas of tenderness. When considering alignment anomalies, tenderness to palpation is a useful criterion to differentiate between dysfunctional misalignment and variations in alignment due to developmental abnormalities, such as a bent spinous process

Any spinal segments exhibiting lack of normal movement (hypomobility), or an increase in normal mobility (hypermobility), should be precisely identified and noted.

Motion palpation" means different things to different people. For some it is a matter of assessing the amount of spinous or transverse process excursion during movement testing; for others it has more to do with the quality of movement, and the end-range feel; and for others yet, it has to do with visualizing vertebral mechanics during side-bending. (Of course, this latter method of assessing vertebral dynamics is not a palpatory method.) I am not one to profess much confidence in the excursion approach to motion palpation, especially in the lumbar spine. The best two examples of this are palpating for the separation and deviation of the spinous processes of the lumbar spine while setting up to perform a side-posture adjustment, alternately raising and lowering the patient's knee while palpating the spinous processes; and the Gillet test for assessing SI motion.

The postural substrate

The tradition in chiropractic of emphasizing global spinal structure seems to begin primarily with Carver, or so it has been written, and has been termed "structuralism," as an alternative to the more ubiquitous approach of emphasizing local findings, which has been called "segmentalism."

The postural substrate is one of the most interesting structural variables with which to work, not because it is known to be more related to back pain than other diagnostic findings - because it isn't - but because the diagnostic information can often be seen from across the room. Information capable of yielding high interexaminer reliability and also capable of being detected non-invasively is not to be overlooked.

Of course, one makes a lot of assumptions in tailoring adjustive vectors for the patient's particular posture, not least among them that it makes a clinical difference when forces are introduced directed contrary to the postural abnormality. There does not appear to be much evidence that thrusting into these spinal convexities, or opening up these spinal concavities, whether understood as segmental lesions or as lateral curvatures, reduces postural distortion in any measurable way. Sometimes it appears that there are postural improvements, but very often there appears to be little or no change.

Nevertheless, we believe there is clinical value in thrusting "as if" one could reduce these curves. This is almost certainly a more reasonable strategy than, say, adjusting with some other intent, such as exaggerating these curves.

Orthopedic testing

The primary purpose of an orthopedic test is to determine what ameliorates, and/or what aggravates musculoskeletal pain; there are hundreds of named orthopedic tests. Apart from documenting the patient's injury or diagnosis, the results of orthopedic testing have immediate implications for adjusting strategies. Although exceptions may arise, as a general rule, lines of drive likely to reproduce the patient's symptoms should be avoided, in favor of those that are likely to reduce them. Suppose, for example, that a patient who has posterior innominate rotation on the left also has a positive Kemp's test on the left (meaning, reproduction of ipsilateral pain on oblique lateral bending). A thrust applied to the left PSIS in side-posture, a fairly typical adjustment for a "PI ilium," could very well reduce the pelvic torsion, but only at the expense of hyperextending the lumbosacral joint, which is contraindicated by the positive Kemp's test. Might another strategy be adopted, to reduced the torsion without reproducing the patient's pain on extension? The answer is yes: the side-posture setup could be modified to include more pre-adjustive flexion, the segmental contact could be made more caudal than usual, the other side of the pelvis could be adjusted as an "AS ilium," a drop-table could be used to limit the amount of extension introduced, padded wedges could be used, etc.

None of this should be interpreted to mean "Thou shalt not adjust in a direction that increases local pain or tenderness"; after all, a person restricted in a certain direction may experience some pain when that restriction is challenged, due to stretching of hypertonic muscles or contractured ligamentous tissues. Nevertheless, at the least, orthopedic tests suggest what directions of thrust are likely to be favorable, and in the case of joint instability, what directions of thrust must be avoided.

Perhaps the biggest exception to the idea of not thrusting when the setup increases pain occurs when the setup at the same time *decreases* distal pain (Mackenzie calls this the "centralization" phenomenon). It is acceptable that local pain increases, at least to some extent, if the flip side is that distal pain and/or neurological symptoms are made less. The converse is also true: a setup that increases distal symptoms (this is called "peripheralization") is a must to avoid, even were it to reduce local pain. In the end, if local pain is increased to the point that the patient is very apprehensive about being adjusted, no good will come of it, even if there has been concurrent centralization. Some other adjustive method will have to be found.

Pre-adjustive tension, which involves bringing the joint in question to its passive end range and applying overpressure without thrusting, is broadly speaking an "orthopedic test." Essentially, the joint is taken to the point of "tension" in an adjustive "set-up" and the patient's response to that position is evaluated. Once again, when mild or moderate local pain or tenderness results, there is no rule dictating how to proceed; the doctor's clinical judgement must prevail. However when significant symptomatology is produced or worsened by a set-up, it is best to avoid thrusting (except, as previously noted, when centralization is apparent).

The following table illustrates that point.

Responses to pre-adjustive tension	Appropriateness of thrusting
Signs of vertebral artery insufficiency	Inappropriate
Neurologic disturbances	Inappropriate
Increased radicular pain	Inappropriate
Severely increased local pain	Inappropriate
Mild to moderately increased local pain	Varies according to severity; more acceptable if distal symptoms reduced
Decreased discogenic or radicular pain	Appropriate, even if local pain increases to some degree

Global range of motion

It is very easy to assess range of motion, not for individual joints, but for regions of the spine, such as lateral flexion of the neck or extension of the lumbar spine. In the frontal plane, we would expect left-right symmetry of range of motion, so that asymmetry indicates regional dysfunction. In the sagittal plane, there is (of course) no notion of symmetry, but we still have the option of comparing the measured amounts with published population means, or better yet, of comparing the ratio of flexion to extension compared to population means.

Having determined inadequacy in a certain direction, the process of determining a line of drive (side of contact, direction of thrust) is very straight-forward: *adjust so as to reduce the global range of motion asymmetry.* We should not be deceived by the simplicity of the "rule," because it protects us from missing the forest for the trees. How frequently would a purely segmental listing lead us to introduce a force which, even were it segmentally appropriate, would be regionally inappropriate? An example would be helpful. Suppose a person has the listing PR for T2, and also is impaired in left lateral flexion of the head and neck to the left. The prone thumb move from right to left at T2 would introduce right lateral flexion, even though what is needed is left lateral flexion for the cervicothoracic region as a whole. In short, *global range of motion* assessment determines the overall reasonability of a procedure that addresses a segmental finding, and may even constitute something of an override where the criteria are inconsistent.

In principle, a segmental finding could override a regional finding, but a lot depends on our confidence in the assessment method. Given the difficulty of consistently reproducing segmental findings, both static and dynamic, it is not obvious under what circumstances they would override a finding as reproducible as a 10^0 lateral bending deficit.

Neurological findings

Patients don't go to "patient finishing school," so they don't typically come in with a set of consistent neurological findings, e.g. a deficient Achilles tendon reflex, difficulty in toe walking, and paresthesia on the lateral aspect of the foot (all signs of an S1 neuropathy). Indeed, that patient may have had problem with heel walking instead, Nevertheless, when a patient does manifest enough signs and symptoms pointing towards a specific nerve root, it is reasonable to focus on that spinal level.

Everything depends on the doctor's ability to discriminate neurologic symptoms from sclerotogenous (referred) pain. How often is pain down the back of the leg considered to be "sciatica," meaning sciatic nerve neuropathy, when in fact posterior leg pain can refer from the sacroiliac, hip, and lumbar spinal joints? Therefore, the appropriateness of addressing a particular body region always depends on the precision of the diagnosis/analysis.

Pain and tenderness

Much has been said in the profession about the unreliability of pain (and other symptoms) as an indicator of pathology, but this author is distinctly unimpressed with these arguments. All organisms, from the first unicellular organisms that arose on earth over 3 billion years ago, to multicellular organisms such as ourselves, have evolved methods of detecting noxious stimuli so as to avoid them. Pain is to Homo sapiens what darkness is to a photosynthetic bacteria: a pointer toward a different and more beneficial direction from which to derive sustenance. I don't believe it has been chiropractic's greatest triumph for some of its practitioners to discover that "pain doesn't matter" after all; luckily most of us still believe that the patient's subjective complaints are somewhat more than a "veil of illusion." I generally (but not always) adjust symptomatic rather than asymptomatic joints. I am not comfortable with another oft-mentioned proviso, to the effect that a hypomobile, pain-free joint is commonly the primary, and a hypermobile, painful joint a mere (non-adjustable) secondary. Although this may occasionally be the case, there is good reason to believe that joints become hypomobile in the first place because there is painful muscle splinting across the joint, at least in acute presentations.

Some clinicians feel that musculoskeletal pain identifies the structure(s) to be adjusted or otherwise treated, whereas others opine that pain identifies areas to be left alone, as putative hypermobile joints, or simply ignored, as "medical" findings. The fact of the matter is, as this author sees it, *pain identifies structures in need of attention.* Although some clinical syndromes are painless or nearly so (e.g., hypertension),it most certainly does not follow that painful conditions are clinically unimportant! The logical fallacy involved is unfortunately commonly seen in chiropractic, but ICT by comparison regards pain as an important indicator, and a very reproducible one at that, of vertebral dysfunction/subluxation states.

Leg checking

Chiropractic leg checking involves determining the relative "length" of the legs - more precisely, determining the relative position of the distal legs - in either a supine or prone patient, by careful observation of the location of the feet. In the Derifield variation of the prone leg check, the feet are also carefully observed with the knees flexed to 90^0. Asymmetry in distal foot positions may be the result of an actual discrepancy in the length of the lower extremities, i.e., structural leg length inequality (LLI); or may result from a postural imbalance, i.e., functional LLI Many chiropractors and allied health professionals feel that LLI, whether structural or functional, may contribute to musculoskeletal pain and degenerative changes, and requires treatment. Moreover, chiropractors believe that functional LLI has diagnostic significance as well, providing evidence of subluxation, generally either intrapelvic (pelvic torsion) or upper cervical (atlas). That granted, reduction of functional LLI serves as an outcome measure, providing evidence of more symmetry in body function and structure.

Manual Muscle Testing

Chiropractors and other Kinesiologists use manual muscle testing as a window into a broad range of purported pathologies: segmentally related or more distant subluxations, allergies, nutritional deficits or needs, learning disabilities, emotional problems, and other entities too numerous (and sometimes too eccentric) to mention. In this context, the strength of a muscle is thought to increase or decrease in response to challenges (diagnostic clinical interventions) of various types and during the course of care, thus providing information on the status of the body's subsystems. The practitioner believes, in assessing muscle strength under a variety of clinical conditions, that he or she is directly communication with the body's nervous system.

In manual muscle testing, the examiner applies force to a muscle or group of muscles while the patient exerts resistance. It is thought by some that different physiological mechanisms are involved according to whether the test is begun by the examiner applying force, before the patient has had a chance to resist (doctor-initiated testing); or the patient first braces by exerting resistance (patient-initiated).

The muscle test amounts to a one-shot, pre-post assessment of a change in muscle strength following a diagnostic intervention, either patient or doctor-initiated. For example, the patient may rotate his neck and head to the left, or touch a point on his abdomen; or the doctor may place a vitamin under the patient's tongue or push a spinous process from right to left. Usually, the baseline muscle is strong and a positive test involves a weakening of the muscle; although sometimes the baseline muscle is weak and a positive test involves strengthening.

Since manual muscle testing is a diagnostic procedure, it must be combined with a thorough history and physical examination to arrive at a clinical impression. It is usually necessary to first identify a previously strong indicator muscle (PSIM), which may in principle be any muscle in the body. The particular muscle chosen happens to be convenient, more than anything else, for the part of the body being diagnosed and the position in which the patient happens to be. For example, the hamstring muscles are very convenient for testing the sacroiliac joints of a prone patient, and the arm flexor group (there is no requirement that one muscle be isolated to be used) for testing points in the inguinal ligament of a supine patient.

Radiographic/radiometric analysis (x-ray line marking)

The rightful role of radiographic analysis in chiropractic has always been controversial, ever since the celebrated incident in which a group of Palmer instructors walked out on B.J. Palmer himself over the issue of introducing radiographic analysis into the curriculum. Everyone agrees that x-rays must be taken to rule out pathology, including contraindications to manipulation, when clinical red flags suggest there may be some; these are called diagnostic x-rays. The main controversy is whether films should be taken for the purpose of obtaining listings; these films, which are taken very differently from one technique system to another, are called analytic x-rays.

X-rays (radiographs) may be taken for either diagnostic purposes, to determine if pathology, including contraindications to adjustive care, is present, or for analytic purposes, to determine listings. By listings, we mean identification of that most traditional of chiropractic pathologies: misalignment – that is, subluxation – of skeletal structures. Analytic X-rays are taken to identify spinal, pelvic, and extremity joint subluxations, as well as to determine reduction or progression of misalignments over time. X-ray line marking methods have been devised to measure distances and angles on radiographs.

Many of the technique systems have developed proprietary patient positioning protocols, X-ray series, and line marking procedures. These are customized relative to each technique system's particular concept of subluxation. Static X-rays of patients neutrally positioned are taken to assess both segmental misalignments and regional disturbances, such as sagittal plane curve abnormalities (hypo- and hyperlordosis, hypo- and hyperkyphosis), and frontal plane lateral curvatures (e.g., scoliosis). Dynamic, or stress X-rays are taken with the patient flexed or extended in the sagittal plane, or side-flexed in the frontal plane, to assess for segmental hypomobility (restriction) or hypermobility (instability). Static and dynamic radiographs, as evaluated by roentgenometric analysis, are thought to help determine appropriate vectors for subluxation correction.

We have heard it said that x-ray line marking is an unreliable procedure, but in our opinion this is not an accurate comment. Many of the line marking systems have shown very high degrees of interexaminer reliability. We have also heard it said that x-ray positioning is an unreliable procedure, meaning we would have little confidence that differences in pre- and post x-rays have to do with bones having moved, rather than differences in the patient positioning. We do not view this as a valid criticism either, there being evidence to the contrary. Ultimately, the problem with x-ray line marking is one of validity: we don't know if any particular measurement tells us something real about the patient. And then, of course, no one has shown that the outcome of care is made better by the clinician having taken x-rays to obtain listings. This problem, in which the clinical utility of a diagnostic/analytic procedure is not yet known, is not exclusive to x-ray line marking, let us say, as compared with leg checking, motion palpation, etc.

ICT allows that there are listings to be derived from x-ray analysis, but adds that in any clinical scenario there must be risk/benefit analysis to see if the films are warranted. X-rays, after all, deliver ionizing radiation to the patient. Apart from this biological cost, there is a considerable financial cost that also must be considered. If an x-ray is considered discretionary, because the patient does not exhibit serious signs and symptoms, then its expense could come out of the same budget that could have funded other health care expenditures that also detect asymptomatic conditions, such as blood pressure examinations (hypertension) and lipid panels (elevated cholesterol levels in the blood). Therefore, *x-rays should never be taken frivolously, just to "see what is going on," or out of exaggerated fears concerning the medicolegal risk of not having taken films.*

Having stated all this, it remains true that radiographic evaluation is a useful diagnostic tool which can be used to assist the practitioner in accurately identifying underlying pathology, anomalies, and spinal listings. Once again: the primary purpose of clinical radiography is to rule out pathology. Once this has been done, the chiropractic practitioner may identify any structural misalignments, congenital anomalies or segmental dysfunction suggested, which may be contributing to the patient's complaints. Appropriate changes are then made to the patient's treatment program, as necessitated by these findings. The use of the computed tomography (CT) scan, magnetic resonance imaging (MRI) and radionuclide bone scans in evaluating spinal problems may also be necessary in certain cases.

Pending better data on the true biohazard that results from the diagnostic/analytic use of ionizing radiation, chiropractic clinicians are urged to show appropriate concern for the biological and economic cost of obtaining x-ray images, and to use the very best radiographic technique they can, when views are deemed necessary, to reduce the ionizing energy to which the patients are exposed.

Thermography

Thermography is a procedure by which the surface temperature of the body can be measured, recorded, and depicted. Although the physiological rationale has been subject to reinterpretation over the years, the prevalent underlying premise is that a difference in surface temperature reflects a difference in vascular flow through the skin, which in turn reflects the state of the nervous system. Specifically, in a state of subluxation, there may be asymmetric left-right paraspinal temperature; or abnormal variation in the temperature of the spinal levels between the sacrum and the atlas; or there may be an abnormal pattern in paraspinal surface temperature as measured over the course of several days.

The dual probe devices employ two thermocouples, one per sensor, and a galvanometer, thus allowing the measurement of left-right paraspinal thermal asymmetry as the unit is applied to the various spinal levels. The single probe devices sense infrared radiation from the skin and produce a digital readout of the temperature at any number of locations, paraspinally and elsewhere. A roller device allows the unit to be kept at a constant distance from the spine. Liquid crystal thermography, in which a thin plastic film placed in contact with the body changes colors in proportion to the surface temperature, is not used much anymore and will not be further described.

Those using dual probe devices, given the finding of left-right thermal asymmetry, are likely to find the warmer side diagnostic of recent subluxation; in essence, evidence of an acute inflammatory response to local tissue damage. By comparison, the cold side may be thought to identify a chronic subluxation, one in which long term tissue damage has resulted in diminished vascularity and blood flow. Given the finding of thermal asymmetry, deciding whether one side is abnormally warm or the other side is abnormally cold must depend on other information, such as the patient's history and other physical examination findings.

Reflex methods

By "reflex technique" we denote technique systems in which observations, palpatory contacts, or other maneuvers relevant to a given part of the body or organ system, can provide information or achieve distant effects at other points -- muscles, organs, joints -- even in cases where no known anatomical or physiological connection can be demonstrated. (Of course, there are many contexts in which the term "reflex" is used in the usual way: deep tendon reflex, somatovisceral reflex, pathological reflex, etc.) Each of the following reflex techniques finds adherents in chiropractic today: iridology, auricular therapy, occipital fiber palpation, organ-muscle relationships, and neurovascular points. Examples of reflex technique include Sacro Occipital Technique and Applied Kinesiology.

The use of reflex methods in chiropractic, where the outcome measure cannot really be explained or rationalized by invoking normal anatomy and physiology as we know it, is obviously very controversial, and will remain controversial into the indefinite future. I can only suggest that the reader remain at least somewhat agnostic on some well-chosen reflex methods.

Notes

1.   Cooperstein R, Gleberzon B. Technique Systems in Chiropractic. Edinburgh: Churchill Livingstone; 2004.
2.   Bergmann T. P.A.R.T.S. joint assessment procedure. Chiropractic Technique 1993;5(3):135-136.

3. Adjustive cornerstones

Manipulation and mobilization

Mobilization is a treatment which passively moves a joint through various points of its available motion up to, but not beyond, the joint's passive end range of motion. It does not move the joint into the paraphysiological space, and does not cause an audible cavitation. The mobilization may be applied singularly or repetitively. This is considered Grades I, II, III, or IV manipulation.

Manipulation, at least as the term is used by chiropractors, is a treatment which employs a thrust to passively move a joint into the paraphysiological space. This is usually accompanied by an audible cavitation, and is considered Grade V motion.

By these distinctions, it is clear that some chiropractic adjustments (discussed immediately below) have the characteristics of mobilization, such as flexion-distraction and pelvic blocking; whereas others have the characteristics of manipulation, such as the P-A thoracic move known as the Carver bridge and A-P thoracic move known as the anterior thoracic. Other chiropractic procedures, including many that qualify as reflex technique procedures, do not obviously resemble either manipulation or mobilization.

Manipulation and adjustment

Careful distinctions have been drawn between the terms "manipulation" and "adjustment." Although pages can and have been written on the subject, the gist of it is that an *adjustment* uses a short lever (such as a transverse or spinous process) to correct a segmental misalignment, whereas a *manipulation* uses longer leverage to increase range of motion, usually in a non-specific sense. Some would add that an adjustment corrects "nerve interference" or in some other way normalizes the nervous system, whereas manipulation is intended only to effect musculoskeletal structures. Although the public may equate the chiropractic adjustment with a high velocity, low amplitude thrust (the type that makes "popping noises" in the spine), the term "adjustment" is a broad term referring to any chiropractic procedure aimed at correcting specific joint dysfunction or subluxation.

To put it bluntly, as some would have it, a manipulation is a poorly-aimed and segmentally non-specific thwack or twisting of the patient's body, whereas an adjustment is a carefully-directed and segmentally specific thrust that removes nerve interference. Manipulation bad, adjustment good. Osteopaths (physiatrists, physical therapists, etc.) "manipulate," and chiropractors "adjust.

There are several problems with this distinction. It is not fair to judge groups other than your own on the basis of stereotypes. Whatever the historical basis for a distinction between osteopathic manipulation and chiropractic adjustment, it would be hard to discern a crucial difference in the methods, judging from both modern and older teaching texts. My copy of Edith Ashmore's 1910 osteopathic text on motion palpation confirms that specificity has always been a consideration for her profession, and appreciation of contemporary figures such as Grieve (physical therapist), Lewit (physiatrist), and Greenman (osteopath) also obviate the hackneyed comparison.

Quite apart from the question of whether the "adjustment" should be considered a proprietary chiropractic method is the clinical question of whether the claimed specificity is actually attainable, and if so, is indeed desirable. The lack of inter-rater reliability that has been found to characterize many chiropractic diagnostic methods, in spite of the practically universal claims of therapeutic effectivity, sketch the following scenario: either diagnostic and/or therapeutic specificity is not substantially related to clinical success, or the universal claims for clinical success are not accurate. In a letter to the editor of JMPT, Haas writes: "If chiropractic can get good results despite poor examiner reliability, then we must consider several possibilities... [Perhaps] we don't have adjusting specificity. Either we are not getting the release in the location that we think we are, therapeusis does not depend as much on the site of the adjustment as we might be led to believe or therapeusis may depend on less localized effects of the adjustment" (Haas, 1990).

Many contemporary chiropractors address vertebral segments while heavily taking into account the local spinal context. These posturalists (better, structuralists) see spinal distortions as frequently, if not usually, multi-segmental, and thus gravitate towards long-lever corrections - even though there is a pronounced tendency towards most of the motion taking place at one motor unit and its immediate neighbors. Their manipulations are as vectored as any thrusts delivered by a segmentalist.

What about the old saw concerning "short-lever adjustments" vs. "long-lever manipulations," another dichotomy in which this issue has been couched? If there is a difference in the clinical outcome of the one type of maneuver compared with the other, then that should be noted and the appropriate conclusions drawn. The scientific parameters that bear on this should receive more attention than the political and economic issues involved, for the sake of the patients if not that of the vested interests. The use of long vs. short levers has to do with the athletic ability of the doctor, the condition and preferences of the patient, and often an intangible sort of aesthetic sense which, like many other opinions on chiropractic technique, is temporarily afforded some viability in the absence of hard facts as to what is actually best to do. The single most-studied chiropractic adjustive procedure, the treatment with the most evidence of effectiveness, the treatment that has become included in healthcare guidelines, is generic spinal manipulation. This makes it very unwise to claim that chiropractors do not perform manipulation. Furthermore, since studies have shown that in the United States, over 94% of all spinal manipulation treatment is performed by chiropractors, we should not exhibit the knee-jerk response, "adjustment good, manipulation bad."

Although ICT certainly respects such traditional distinctions, it also recognizes that the evidence is not in yet on how and whether specific, short levered interventions produce a different outcome compared with longer-levered, less specific (regional) interventions. One thing seems certain: deciding between the two approaches ought to be a matter of desired outcome, not a matter of philosophy. That means it is perfectly acceptable for a chiropractor to manipulate to increase range of motion, if that is the goal of care; therefore the term "manipulation" should not be used as a code word to describe bad chiropractors who function like allopaths.

Moreover, ICT recognizes that since certain problems are best understood as regional in nature, that clinically appropriate intervention may well include a regional approach, like having the "punishment fit the crime." Let's suppose a hunchback named Quasimodo shows up at our chiropractic clinic complaining of pain between the shoulder blades. How relevant would it be to his problem, to decide that he has a"PR" of T4, perhaps after 10 minutes of careful and specific palpation, when in fact his real listing is hunchbackism? And, from a treatment point of view, wouldn't the compassionate approach involve finding a way to flatten the hump, as compared with attempting to rotate T4? As a counterexample, we may consider the case of torticollis, which this author commonly finds associated with a specific rotational misalignment in the upper cervical spine. That should best be addressed by a segmentally-specific, carefully controlled thrust -- that is, an adjustment in the classic sense of the term.

When a thrust or other manual intervention is delivered that is likely to affect multiple segments, whether to address a lateral curvature or abnormal sagittal curve, it may be every bit as directionally specific as an adjustment. I would call such interventions "vectored manipulations." Again, let the punishment fit the crime.

The table below summarizes some of the relationships we have been describing, comparing and contrasting what are termed the "historical" (mostly philosophical) and "contemporary" (mostly biomechanical) points of view concerning adjustment, mobilization, and manipulation.

	Adjustment	**Mobilization**	**Manipulation**
Historical point of view	More specific and highly skilled than mobilization or manipulation. The procedure which reduces subluxation.	Unspecific, gross movement of joints used as a treatment by DOs, MDs, or PTs.	Unspecific, gross movement of joints used as a treatment by DOs, MDs, or PTs.
Contemporary point of view	A wide variety of manual and mechanical chiropractic procedures.	Movement applied within the physiologic range of joint motion.	A thrust procedure which moves a joint past the physiologic range of motion

Mechanical advantage

Consider, if you will, the following metaphor. A clock is slow by 5 minutes, and the time may be corrected by rotating either the hour, minute, or second hand through some amount of arc. One may elect to rotate the hour hand through 2.5 degrees, using a relatively large amount of force; or, using substantially less force (1/60 as much), rotate the minute hand through an arc of 30 degrees. Finally, one could turn the second hand 5 full times around the clock face, taking it through a full 1800 degrees, but requiring only 1/3600 as much force as that required using the hour hand to correct the time. At the risk of oversimplification, the given amount of work required to "adjust" the time may be accomplished using either a large force over a small distance (a short-lever correction), or a lesser force applied over a longer distance (a long-lever correction). This clock metaphor illuminates some of the choices that are to be made in choosing particular avenues of approach to the spinal subluxation syndromes. For example, a thrust on the sacral apex has a much longer lever than a thrust on the sacral base. A small doctor may prefer the longer levers, or any doctor may prefer them for larger patients. The shorter levers, on the other hand, allow more control over what exactly is going on. Nothing is "right" or "wrong" in this, it's a question of the cost/benefit ratio of the different options.

Rehabilitation procedures

The doctor must decide if the goal of care is mostly short term crisis intervention, mostly for the purpose of alleviating the patient's pain (over 90% of chiropractic patients list pain as their primary complaint), mostly long term maintenance/wellness/preventive/rehabilitative (the terms overlap) care, or something in-between. Rehabilitation procedures are largely directed at chronic patients, who account for the bulk of health care costs in our society, at least when it comes to spine-related complaints. These are not adjustive procedures *per se*, but they serve as a useful adjunct to adjustive procedures. Although the concept of "holding an adjustment" seems a little quaint these days, lacking an operational definition, the idea behind it is simple enough and well-founded: we must look beyond what listing the patient has, and determine not only that, but what type of patient has the listing. Is the patient in good or bad health? Is the patient fit as a fiddle, or deconditioned? Correcting subluxations in an unhealthy patient and leaving it at that is like applying a fresh coat of paint over a peeling surface, without having prepared the old surface to receive a new coat of paint.

Patient selection

The most important three factors in predicting the outcome using a specific adjustive procedure, for a specific condition, upon a specific patient are: *patient selection, patient selection,* and *patient selection.* It almost goes without saying that a procedure useful for a given patient may be worse than useless for another, that *it therefore makes no sense to judge the relative merits of various techniques independently of the patients.* Spinal surgeons frequently state that the outcome depends on the right doctor doing the right surgery on the right patient at the right time – should it be any different for chiropractic adjustive procedures.

The text is not written, the one that would tell us what chiropractic technique procedure has been proven optimal under various clinical circumstances, and yet we are required to forge ahead with treatment while the evidence base accumulates. In the meantime, we will have to use common sense, clinical experience, and the evidence such as it is to choose among the various treatment options. And so we might use low force methods on patients with osteoporosis, drop-table methods on patients unable to lie in side-posture, and padded wedges on a low back pain patient who is terrified of popping noises from the spine.

Doctor selection

Doctor selection is also very important. Let's face it, chiropractic adjusting is on some level an athletic ability. No sooner would I expect every chiropractor to be equally adept at every procedure there is than I would expect any person to be equally talented at figure skating. It may be that the outcome using a particular procedure may have more to do with who is doing it than with the procedure itself.

Apart from differences in individuals' innate psychomotor abilities, at any moment injuries could arise that put limitations on what the doctor can and can't do. One only hopes that a doctor, forced to alter his or her adjusting style due to an injury, can find alternative techniques that are believed to be equally effective; and it is a good idea for all doctors to have developed a variety of methods in which they have confidence, just for such a rainy day. Doctors must also apply the same principles of ergonomics to their own adjusting methods that they would apply to their patient's occupational exposures. They must prevent injuries to their own bodies, especially resulting from their daily practice of chiropractic, if they are to continue to be able to administer chiropractic care to their patients.

Joint kinematics

Clinical experience suggests that spinal manipulation requires less force and achieves better outcomes when the thrust is applied in accordance with the normal kinematics for the joint concerned. That, of course, involves knowing the typical coupling patterns for the different articulations of the spine. One example here might be worth a thousand words. Lateral flexion of the lower cervical spine is accompanied by ipsilateral body rotation. Therefore, the traditional modified rotary break adjustment, which involves laterally flexing the supine patient's neck to the side, and then rotating the head and the neck to the other side, imposes a non-physiological prestress on the joints of the lower cervical spine. Is this harmful, or does it generate a bad outcome? Not necessarily, but the anatomical considerations suggest that it would make sense to avoid extremely "unphysiological" setups.

For the example given, perhaps the neck could be kept closer to the midline of the table, rather than being flexed markedly to the side. It is reasonable to suppose gaining access to a joint's "paraphysiological space" (that range of motion beyond what the patient can access through the normal movements of daily life, accessible only through a manipulative thrust) is likely to be safer, short and long term, if proper joint kinematics are observed. Lewit, perfectly aware of the anatomical considerations, nevertheless finds value in what he would call "asynkinetic" set-ups (i.e., patient pre-stressing that involves atypical coupling patterns) because he thinks they increase the specificity of his thrust. While we await data on matters such as these, we all have to do what we think is best; ICT believes it best that our understanding of physiological coupling patterns impact upon our adjusting methods.

In a related vein, if the patient can be pre-positioned by pre-stressing the various joints so as to reverse his or her presenting distortion, then the manipulative thrust gains access to the paraphysiological space in a manner least likely to incur damage. To put it simply, patients may be pre-positioned to ameliorate their usual distorted posture, and thus brought toward this "corrected" direction by adjustment in accordance with the normal kinematics for the spinal-pelvic area in question. As an example, a patient with a right thoracic spine curvature could be pre-positioned with a left spinal curvature, prior to the doctor thrusting, whether using a prone or supine setup. Another example: a patient with exaggerated thoracic kyphosis could be adjusted prone, whereas another patient with a diminished ("saucered") thoracic curve could be adjusted in the supine position with the thorax held off the table by the doctor while the thrust is being delivered.

AS-IF Adjusting

There is clinical value in thrusting "as if" one could reduce these curves. This is almost certainly a more reasonable strategy than, say, adjusting with some other intent, such as exaggerating these curves. However transient the altered vertebral positions, in the process there is stretching of contracted tissues, approximation of distended tissues, reduction of fibrosis and possibly inflammation, interruption of positive feedback loops, improvement of muscle synergism, enhanced neurological function, reduced facilitation, and maybe more. In the act of setting the bones in motion toward a more neutral and probably optimal position, one anticipates an ultimate normalization in function by means of increased flexibility, range, and smoothness of motion. Although we do occasionally note some reduction of lateral curvatures, which usually corresponds to a reduction in patient symptoms, we would generally use this strategy even when it is unrealistic, as in the case of idiopathic juvenile scoliosis, to expect much, if any, structural change.

It takes a lot of practice to develop the art of vertebral manipulation, a lot of emotional tranquility, to learn this art of silent conversation with the patient's unconscious neuromuscular control mechanisms. It also takes a thorough knowledge of normal kinematics to learn how to make one's corrections by means of proper pre-positioning rather than by using excessive force, so that the joints are likely to gap and sheer in exactly the optimal way. We take into account the nature of the movements that normally occur when the patient engages in active motion.

Assisted and resisted adjustments

Nomenclatural rules or kinematics?

As we have stated above, the terminological convention by which we list the superior bone should not imply that the underlying biomechanical fault resides in the one segment rather than the other, insofar as the subluxation occurs in the joint between the two. Furthermore, there is no a priori reason to suppose that when a clinician attempts to reduce the subluxation by applying a thrust, that the force which is applied moves a segment with respect to the one below, any more than with respect to the segment above. Cineradiography has demonstrated that a manipulative thrust introduces a damped disturbance into the spine which extends to several motor units both above and below the point of contact, although it affects the immediately adjacent articulations the most. It's one thing to list L4 with respect to L5, but quite another to suppose that a contact on L4 affects primarily the joint between the two (as opposed to L3-4). Chiropractors have put a lot of work in recent years into trying to understand which articulations are primarily affected by the adjustive procedures they use, and have begun to deploy a new terminology to discuss their findings. This is discussed below.

Although by convention we *list a vertebra* as being subluxated (misaligned, fixated, or both) in relation to the segment below, that does not mean that an adjustive thrust necessarily primarily affects *the joint below*. It all depends on the doing. The "assisted-resisted" terminology is gradually taking root among the chiropractic colleges. Although we cannot go into the intricacies here, especially since much of it remains somewhat speculative at the current time, the basic point seems well-taken and is worth noting.

Let us provide an example. When the doctor sets up to perform a thumb move on the prone patient at the T2 level, stabilizing on the patient's head and neck above, clearly, the primary articulation effected is T1-2. The reason? The main action must take place between the doctor's two hands, not below the contact hand. If this does not seem obvious, then consider what happens when you wring a wet bath towel between your two hands to expel the water. Doesn't the water pour out between your hands, as compared with the ends of the towel?

Adjustments that produce movement above the contact hand have been called "*resisted*," and those that produce movement below the contact hand (e.g., side-posture adjustment of L4 with pocket-to-pocket stabilization) have been called "*assisted*."[1] Chiropractic Technique 1992;4(4):117-123.), but our point in bringing up the matter is not really to fret about the terminology, but to communicate the point that every chiropractor must

---

[1] 1. Good CJ. An analysis of diversified (lege artis) type adjustments based upon the assisted-resisted model of intervertebral motion unit prestress. Chiropractic Technique 1992;4(4):117-123.

carefully consider what exact joints are likely to be affected by the maneuver he or she is considering, and to modify those procedures as necessary to bring about the desired result.

Structural findings

No claim is made that utilizing the principles of kinematic adjusting and vectored pre-positioning guarantees "correction" or even substantial improvement in abnormal curvatures - although sometimes it seems that it does. Rather, it is the case that these principles increase the probability that the joints will at minimum be substantially moved, and that soft tissues which have entered into chronic contractures (on the concave sides of abnormal curves) will in fact be lengthened. The principle involved here is that the doctor should adjust *as if to change* curves and curvatures, even if changes are not likely to be forthcoming.

Segmental intervention, indications

When a particular patient is best understood as suffering from subluxation in the narrow sense of the term, meaning *segmental misalignment*, then the patient should be addressed as such. A specific thrust should be delivered, using a line of drive likely to realign that segment in relation to contiguous structures. If the diagnosis had more to do with movement restriction, then the thrust would be designed to restore movement in whatever degrees of freedom (among the 6 possibilities) the functional unit is restricted. [more to come]

Regional intervention, indications

This author once heard a radio announcer say "regional problems demand regional solutions." The radio personality was talking about certain banking problems afflicting parts of the United States, but the remarks were very relevant to this paragraph, that I knew I would be writing later in the day. If the patient's posture is abnormal, or if there are problems with global ranges of motion, or both; then the patient should be addressed accordingly.

A fresh look at the adjustive technique schema

For many decades in chiropractic adjustive procedures have been characterized in a standard way according to their basic elements: patient position, doctor's stance, tissue pull, segmental contact point, contact point, and line of drive. Although the schema has shown remarkable staying power, it is starting to appear a little frayed around the edges. It is time to take a fresh look at it, reflecting on how new research findings impact upon its utility. Although there is some value in having a standard format to describe adjustive procedures, the schema bears the imprint of biomechanical assumptions that require reinterpretation in the light of new knowledge. Doing so could simplify learning adjustive procedures, and may ultimately improve the outcome of chiropractic care. Let us discuss each of these parameter in turn, with particular emphasis on research developments that challenge the conventional wisdom.

Table 1. The traditional adjustive procedure schema

Parameter	Abbreviation
Patient position	PP
Doctor's stance	DS
Contact point	CP
Segmental contact point	SCP
Torque	Torque
Tissue pull	TP
Stabilization	SH
Line of drive (or correction)	LOD (or LOC)

Patient position

All adjustive setup descriptions must include a preferred position for the patient: supine, prone, seated, standing, on all fours, or side-lying. On the other hand, very few technique manuals or textbooks account for patient variations that may take precedence over the doctor's preferred style, or even preclude it. What, for example, happens when a patient simply can not tolerate side-lying, or becomes very apprehensive when placed supine for an anterior thoracic maneuver? Common sense dictates that the adjustive style and thus patient position must be modified in such cases, and yet it is rare to find backup plans included within the traditional adjustive procedure schema. Modern doctors of chiropractic had best worry not only about what listing the patient has, but what type of patient has the listing.

Doctor's stance

Fencer's stance (aka scissors stance), straight-away stance, standing at the head of the table (favoring one corner or not: all are acceptable, depending on the mechanics of the adjustment to be accomplished. On the other hand, rules calling for standing on the left or right side of the table, owing to the side of the segmental contact, might best yield to more basic considerations, such as handedness. Not surprisingly, right-handed people instinctively stand on prone patient's left side, no doubt to get the dominant hand closer to the patient. Likewise, they tend to stand on the supine patient's right side while performing the anterior thoracic adjustment, so as deploy the dominant hand in applying the force to the patient's crossed arms. One supposes left-handed doctors would assume reversed stance sides, in accordance with having a left dominant arm, but I can not say with confidence that I have seen this tendency. According to Peterson (personal communication) there are circumstances, in supine adjusting, when it becomes necessary to develop competency with both hands; as when unilateral contacts are used to generate rotation.

Contact point

It is fair to say that chiropractors have duly considered that there are many ways to use the hands to apply forces to patients for thrusting and other adjustive procedures. The traditional technique schema does not take into account that the choice of contact point should involve doctor considerations at least as much as it does purely mechanical characteristics. For example, a doctor with carpal tunnel syndrome might want to avoid using a double thenar contact, for fear of aggravating the condition by chronically hyperextending the wrist. Looking at the thoracic spine alone, the various traditional contacts include the double thenar, the Carver bridge (aka double hypothenar), the single-hand contact (aka reinforced pisiform or hypothenar), and the crossed pisiform (aka double transverse). (See figure 1). Although there is little reason to suppose any of these contacts has a significant therapeutic advantage over another, there are some differences from an ergonomic point of view. The double thenar contact, used over and over, may eventually result in a wrist sprain due to loading the wrist in hyperextension; at the other end of the ergonomic spectrum is the Carver bridge, which possesses the same advantage as keyboards that are designed to protect the typist's wrist by keeping the hands partially supinated. The traditional technique schema is not flexible enough to accommodate such considerations.

Segmental contact point

The discussion of "contact point" would be far less arcane if the chiropractic profession had settled upon anatomical locations that made more sense, even allowing for the very significant fact that the doctor actually contacts soft tissue, not bone. How, after all, how *could* a doctor hope to make contact with a mammilary process or lamina-pedicle junction? One would be hard-pressed to come up with spinal structures more difficult to imagine contacting, even with the pointiest pisiform ever! Then, of course, there is the matter of soft tissue. There has been surprisingly little discussion of how muscle and myofascial tissues complicate the matter of placing the the doctor's hands in a location likely to achieve the intended impact on joints. After all, the effective force or pressure landing on a segmental contact must be effected by the stiffness or lack thereof the intervening soft tissue, as well as the friction between the skin and the underlying osseous structures. According to Herzog et al "as the forces during spinal manipulative treatment increase, so does the contact area; therefore, much of the total treatment force is taken up by non-target-specific tissues" (1). When all is said and done, the data suggest that the effective force imparted to a thoracic transverse force, using a reinforced hypothenar is a very small fraction of the total force produced: "The average peak total force was 238.2 N. The average peak local force over a target area of 25 mm^2 was 5 N, indicating that global measures of loading vastly overestimate the local effective forces at the target site (1), Moreover, "The peak pressure point moved, on average, 9.8 mm during the course of the manipulation" (1). Bereznick et al also found that the hand was displaced from the segmental contact point during a thrusting procedure (2). Hessel et al (3) found that two clinicians had great difficulty landing a thrust on the PSIS, winding up invariably on the sacrum. We are not surprised by these findings, that adjustive specificity may be difficult to attain. Since many thrusting techniques extend the elbows from an initially flexed position, any force delivered in a non-perpendicular manner *must* move the hands away from their pre-adjustive position on the patient. Finally, Perle et al (4) have shown that subtle changes in the way the hand is used may have a substantial impact on the location and amount of force delivered.

Torque

The concept of torque is not holding up very well in the chiropractic technique and research worlds. It is hardly, if at all, included in testing at the National Board level. Harrison et al (5) criticized the typical usage of torque in chiropractic adjustments, although Herzog (6) felt Harrison himself had in turn misused the term. It is reasonable to assume spinal adjustments can rotate vertebra, and that the term torque (as the cross product of lever arm and applied force) can be used to describe such forces as would impart vertebral rotation. For example, a P to A thrust on a transverse process is likely to turn the vertebra around the Y axis of the body. Unfortunately, chiropractors most commonly use the term torque to describe how the hand might be spun while delivering a thrust, so as to impart that same spin to the contacted bone. That is the aspect of "torque" that is not holding up well: there is a world of difference between one object impacting another object off its axis of rotation so as to make it spin, and what happens when a spinning object strikes a stationary object. It is unlikely that spinning the hand on the flesh above the intended segmental contact does anything other than stretch the skin, thus comprising a special form of "tissue pull," another term whose significance is very debatable (see below). The most peculiar application of the torque concept in chiropractic is probably in the toggle-recoil adjustment of atlas, in which the doctor's spinning hand is applied parallel to the length of the transverse process, as though it were a torque wrench of some kind.

Tissue pull

It is reasonable to attempt displacing intervening soft tissue (some would say remove tissue slack) to get one's hand closer to the intended bony contact under the skin. It is also reasonable to define the direction of tissue pull, generally in the same direction as the intended thrust to follow. The problems that arise have to do with variation in patient's skin elasticity. Suppose, for example, that the T7 transverse processes are the target for a double hypothenar (Carver bridge) style intervention. The principle of tissue pull requires that the adjustor place the hypothenar contacts somewhat caudad to the target, then slide up to the T7 level to attain the segmental contact point. Since some patients will have very elastic skin, and others relatively inelastic skin, it is not clear from which start point the adjustor should begin the inferior to superior tissue pull. Locating the T7 target is challenging enough without complicating the matter by contacting the spine inferior to it, then tugging the skin some unknown amount so as to wind up exactly on T7. As an alternative, It is possible to work the hypothenar contacts into the skin at the location of the intended target, a procedure that might be called "tissue burrowing." It is reasonable to assume this would ensure greater accuracy in attaining the intended target.

Stabilization (aka indifferent) hand

It is deeply embedded in chiropractic technique that one hand can be defined as the primary mover, while the other hand somehow "stabilizes" other spinal or pelvic structures to increase the specificity of the adjustment. On the other hand, scrutinizing various adjustive procedures quickly reveals that the so-called stabilization hand is often also cast as an agent of vertebral movement, either reinforcing the contact hand or moving other structures just as surely as the so-called contact hand. Grieve ((7), p 557) provides a very eloquent description pertinent to cervical manipulation. He very ably describes how subtle changes in the method determine which joints are primarily affected, and how they are affected by *each* hand. Taking the joint to full tension and emphasizing the contact hand (Grieve calls it the "executive hand") shears the contacted side. On the other hand, applying a slightly slower thrust to a less-then fully tensioned joint, while using the contralateral hand to aggressively distract and side-flex toward the contact hand, primarily gaps the side opposite the contact hand. Indeed, in this case the so-called stabilization hand is more rightfully considered the contact (executive) hand.

Line of drive / line of correction

Line of drive and line of correction are usually used interchangeably to denote the vector the clinicians attempts to employ in delivering a manipulative thrust. Research done at the Canadian Memorial Chiropractic College challenges the conventional wisdom that the line of drive makes a difference, by showing that non-perpendicular forces dissipate the effective force delivered to the spine. In so many words, any force delivered oblique to the spine just stretches the skin. As Bereznick et al (2) put it: "efforts to apply an oblique force during thoracic manipulation may be wasted effort. For example, applying a force on a 45^0 angle from normal to the skin will reduce the magnitude of the resultant force experienced by the underlying vertebra to 70.7% of the applied force . . . This clinician would be spending 29.3% of their effort transmitting loads elsewhere creating deformation of the skin and producing a general translation of the entire patient along the table."

In conclusion, the adjustive procedure schema is looking a little frayed around its edges. In its present form, it may be more useful at generating multiple choice questions than teaching chiropractic students how to adjust. Its rows contain many implicit assumptions that belie the data coming out of the laboratories that are researching spinal manipulation. There is no major harm in using this concise format for describing how the doctor and patient would be positioned, and what each hand would be doing in a rough sense, at least as the first approximation of the skill to be learned by a chiropractic student. However, at some point we must realize and remember the following:

- It is difficult, if not impossible, to accurately deliver a force to a small spinal structure, in part due to soft tissue influences.
- The practice of tissue pull may further decrease the accuracy of hand placement.
- Even with accurate delivery, only a small fraction of the total force applied or pressure created lands on the target.
- Non-perpendicular lines of drive dissipate force and worsen accuracy, while simply stretching the skin.
- Recommendations for doctor and patient position must be subject to modification, taking into account specific doctor and patient characteristics.
- The so-called stabilization hand is usually more aptly considered "the

other contact hand."

- The concept of torque, at least insofar as it refers to a spinning contact hand, should be abandoned.

Byfield's excellent book on chiropractic manipulation (8) entirely bypasses the technique schema as we know it, and yet still manages to wonderfully describe and depict how chiropractic adjustments are done.

Note for discussion of adjustive schema

1.   Herzog W, Kats M, Symons B. The effective forces transmitted by high-speed, low-amplitude thoracic manipulation. Spine 2001;26(19):2105-10; discussion 2110-1.
2.   Bereznick DE, Ross JK, McGill SM. The frictional properties at the thoracic skin-fascia interface: implications in spine manipulation. Clin Biomech (Bristol, Avon) 2002;17(4):297-303.
3.   Hessel BW, Herzog W, Conway PJW, al e. Experimental measurement of the force exerted during spinal manipulation using the Thompson technique. J Manipulative Physiol Ther 1990;13(8):448-453.
4.   Perle SM, Kawchuk GN. Pressures generated during spinal manipulation and their association with hand anatomy. J Manipulative Physiol Ther 2005;28(4):e1-7.
5.   Harrison DD, Colloca CJ, Troyanovich SJ, Harrison DE. Torque: an appraisal of misuse of terminology in chiropractic literature and technique. J Manipulative Physiol Ther 1996;19(7):454-62.
6.   Herzog W. Torque: an appraisal of misuse of terminology in chiropractic literature and technique. J Manipulative Physiol Ther 2000;23(4):298-9.
7.   Grieve G. Common Vertebral Joint Problems. 2 ed. Edinburgh London Melbourne and New York: Churchill Livingstone; 1988.
8.   Byfield D. Chiropractic Manipulative Skills. Edinburgh: Elsevier Churchill Livingstone; 2005.

4. The physiology of standing

The mechanism of standing

Standing is much more difficult than it seems. Careful observation of subjects who did not know they were being observed has revealed that during relaxed standing they constantly shifted their weight from one leg to the other, about twice per minute (Smith, 1953).

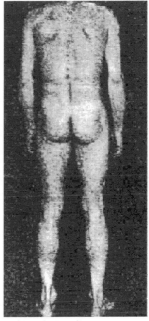

Relaxed standing

Several advantages accrue from this oscillatory performance:

• Tissue fluid is imbibed into and expressed from intervertebral disks and other cartilaginous structures, such as the menisci of the knees.

• Synovial fluid is produced in increased quantity.

• At any moment in time, ½ of the musculature that is involved in the maintenance of balance is relaxed.

Let us recall that the sagittal plane gravity line passes anterior to the ankle, and that tendencies to sway forward and backward are checked mainly by the posterior ankle ligaments and tibialis anterior, respectively. Even during relaxed standing there is constant activity of the soleus muscle (and gastrocnemius, to a lesser extent) to maintain balance. It is necessary to periodically shift weight to relax the balancing muscles, so that fatigue does not develop and compromise the integrity of the balancing system (Joseph, 1960, p. 54).

In addition to this macroscopic left/right weight shifting, there are more subtle swaying motions both to and fro and left to right. Joseph (1960, p.17) describes these sway patterns in normal subjects: "Swaying in both the sagittal and frontal planes does occur and varies in different individuals. The backward and forward swaying is more marked than the side to side swaying, and takes place about the transverse axes of the ankle joints, so that the top of the head moves more than any other part of the body." The extent of this swaying in 43 subjects aged 18-30 was as follows: 41.7 +/- 1.6 mm in the to and fro, and 29.7 +/-1.8 mm from side to side. The effects were greater in old people, and in young women as well.

The magnitude of the sway increases, but the frequency decreases, during prolonged standing. There are actually 2 oscillations in at-ease standing: a relatively slow and large to-and-fro movement, superimposed on a series of smaller to-and-fro oscillations. These same motion patterns were detected by Jansen and Nansel (Jansen et al, JMPT1990;13(7):361-9.) using an alternative quad scale technology that tracked fluctuations in the body's center of gravity. It is likely that this swaying mechanism complements the alternating slouch patterns in maintaining joint fluidity and ameliorating fatigue. It should go without saying that the finding that standing sway patterns are normal physiology calls into question certain chiropractic examination procedures that focus on "AP" and "lateral" sway as diagnostic categories of sacroiliac dysfunction.

Pathology of standing

The dynamic quality to the act of standing immediately suggests a mechanism by which long-term postural asymmetries may develop. Although at any one moment in time we would expect more weight to be borne by one of the limbs, we nevertheless presume that there is no long-term tendency for one of the limbs to be more favored in this manner. In other words, the total amount of weight borne by each leg would average out to be 50%, even though at any one moment in time it is likely to be very different from 50%. It could be said that we go through life standing in slouched postures, constantly switching between left and right poses. It's as though we were "sitting on ourselves" (on one side of the body) in the standing position.

Now let us suppose that by some means one side of slouch becomes favored. This could be the result of an accident, handedness and footedness patterns, an occupational risk, a certain attitudinally-related body language, acquired or congenital anatomic asymmetry, or possibly some other factor. For example, let us suppose either a subluxation of the sacrum (as did Dr. Hugh Logan) or an obliquity of the pelvis (as did the Kendalls). If these postural aberrations were to take origin during the growing years, anything less than a complete return to symmetry would certainly result in irreversible structural distortion, through a long-term process of bony remodeling.

Apart from the effects on osseous, ligamentous, and muscular structures, there would be complementary neurological sequella, in terms of learning to accept these asymmetric postures as "normal." Proprioceptive perception of distortion and/or reflexive muscular response to it do not succeed in reversing this process, so that we learn to accommodate to distorted frames. In the end, one of the standing slouch positions becomes - literally - "second nature."

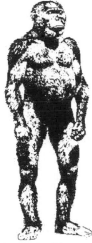

Since asymmetric musculoskeletal structures are likely to experience osteoarthritic breakdown at different rates, one supposes that individuals becoming habituated to characteristic slouch patterns may accelerate their own musculoskeletal breakdown. At the same time, given the obvious observation that such patterns are ubiquitous, we presume some developmental advantage to some degree of asymmetry in musculoskeletal structure, whether to accommodate the division of labor between the left and right sides of the brain, footedness and handedness patterns, or both. At a time in hominid evolutionary history when our ancestors tended to die young by modern standards (pre-Homo sapiens hominids rarely lived beyond 30 years), one assumes the advantages of structural and functional asymmetry outweighed the disadvantages of accelerated arthritic breakdown. In other words, we died of starvation, trauma, disease, or predation long before arthritis became much of a concern. By comparison, in modern times,

Australopithecus afarensis, c. 3.5 million years ago. Walked bipedally but wasn't very bright.

life extension now permits us to live long enough for asymmetry to pose a health threat. Enter the chiropractor: the specialist in helping Homo sapiens cope with the musculoskeletal consequences of life extension. Chiropractic care may be thought of as geriatric care for patients older than teenagers, from this point of view.

Standing as portrayed in art

Relatively early Greek statues tend to portray standing figures in a very symmetric way. As generations of sculptors went by, their works became more asymmetric, as if to say the Greeks understood that humans were more perfect – were, in a way, more human – when they stood in an asymmetric posture. Most of the weight would be borne on one leg, whereas the other leg would show foot flare, and a flexed knee and hip. The figure shows increasing modernity, left to right.

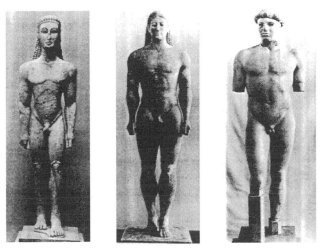

The *Spear Thrower* is considered one of the great works of western art. Inspection shows most of the weight is borne on the right leg, with the left leg turned out and used more for balancing. The lowering of the left hip results partially from posterior innominate rotation, but more importantly, from the postural habit of flexing the right hip and knee. Moreover, pronation of the right foot adds to the lowering of the ipsilateral side of the pelvis.

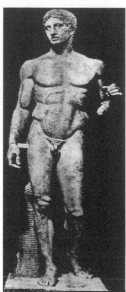

The Spear Thrower

It is commonly believed that foot flare is related to an IN ilium. Usually, the explanation that follows states that as the ilium moves medially on the sacrum, the acetabular facing becomes more lateral, thus causing foot flare. Unfortunately, this is unlikely to be true, since the amount of movement available to the SI joint is not adequate to explain the typical 10 degrees or more of foot flare that might be seen. It is much more logical to see foot flare as resulting from external hip rotation, with a possible contribution from the subtalar joint, rather than the consequence of a putative SI movement or misalignment of some kind. Then, foot flare would reflect a postural habit that in turn reflects a lowered hemipelvis on the side of the flared foot, as the sculptures show. Our hypothesis is that the lowered pelvis is related to a posteriorly related ilium, and the associated hip and knee flexion that goes along with that, as Hugh Logan explained.

Since the ilium is very likely to track medially when it moves posteriorly, given the shape and facing of the SI joint, to say that foot flare tends to be associatred with posterior ilium rotation is tantamount to saying it is associated with medial ilium movement, the so-called "IN ilium." Thus, it is possible to deduce foot flare as related to IN ilium starting in a novel way: not as directly related to SI movement, and a changed acetabular facing, but rather directly related to external hip rotation as it accompanies pelvic torsion. Then, the foot flare relates to the IN component of what amounts to a PI-IN movement of the ilium, to use standard Gonstead terminology for the moment.

Standing and the gait mechanism

The behavior of the torso during walking has been well-studied, although the exact role of the sacroiliac joints in this remains somewhat unclear. As is discussed in detail in chapters to come, the innominate bones are capable of rotating in opposite directions around an axis transversely through the symphysis pubis, one rotating anteriorward and the other posteriorward. Although we later discuss this as a matter of interinnominate subluxation, in the classic chiropractic sense of the term, in this present discussion we are talking about the normal kinematics of walking, in which the innominate bones engage in the same opposed rotation. During walking, the innominate bones oscillate between anterior and posterior rotation, in a reciprocal and opposed manner. The frequency is 2 oscillations per step, defined as the interval from toe-off to heel-strike. The innominate is anteriorly rotated at toe-off, becomes posteriorly rotated during early swing phase, rotates anteriorly later in swing phase, and comes to rest posteriorly rotated at heel-strike.

At heel-strike the pelvis is inferior on the ipsilateral side, and the lumbar spine possesses a lateral curvature that is ipsilaterally convex. These are the essential parameters of the basic distortion, as Dr. Logan termed it, that was previously described, clearly implying that slouched standing postures are nothing other than habitual trunk postures that normally occur during walking. In effect, the trunk is "still walking" while the extremities are retracted to the neutral position. More precisely, the slouched standing posture corresponds to early heel-strike, before much of the body weight has been transferred to the striking heel.

Of course, if slouched standing were to be regarded as a frozen phase of gait, then the flip-side of the proposition would be to regard gait as a displaced static pose. In fact, the classic description of walking was rendered by Steindler as follows: "a series of catastrophes narrowly averted." We extend the leg forward during walking in order to avoid crashing to the ground once the center of gravity has been displaced anteriorly. Abnormalities in the gait mechanism are analogs of faulty postures. The marriage of slouched stance as a static gait and a clumsy gait as dynamized slouch completes the analogy.

It is illustrative to perform a little experiment. Let the reader clasp his or her hands, noting which thumb is over the other; then, reverse this "hand posture" so that the other thumb is on top. A great majority of individuals find this reversed posture very uncomfortable, and a few are almost incapable of even attaining it in less than 10 seconds. Is it too much to suggest that we become equally at home with one direction of relaxed standing, so that the mirror image stance is distinctly uncomfortable?

From a clinical chiropractic point of view, it becomes a question of noting which stance is habitual and customary, so that a series of listings ranging from the foot to the midthoracic spine is generated. Which of these posturally-generated listings are optimal to adjust in a given office visit is another story, but the menu of possibilities can often be seen from several yards away.

The chapters that follow track this basic distortion, from its roots in the gait

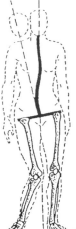

mechanism to its consequences as mechanical distortion and symptoms of musculoskeletal origin. As is customary, we proceed from the low back, to the thoracic spine, and finally to the cervical spine. This presentation is largely confined to the axial skeleton, and thus we are remiss in not attending more to the pelvic and shoulder girdles. We will have to ameliorate this problem in a future revision of this text. For many patients, there could be no thought of addressing a cervicothoracic complaint without dealing with possible shoulder (i.e., glenouhumeral and scapulocostal) problems, nor could we adequately address lumbopelvic problems without taking into account the contribution made to the overall problem by the lower extremities.

Although we have the basic distortion, what may be called *primary pelvic torsion*, on the radar screen, we must stay on the lookout for the exceptions that prove the rule: the patients whose spinal distortions are not coherent, and the patients whose problems are better understood from a segmental point of view. Moreover, we must consider the possibility torsion is *secondary*: that a patient may have a structural asymmetry in leg lengths; indeed, probability, given the finding by several investigators that as many as half of normal subjects, and a larger proportion of symptomatic subjects, have anatomic leg length inequality of a quarter inch or more. Indeed, when chiropractors perform leg checks, whether to infer pelvic distortion or atlas misalignment (the usual clinical intention), the possibility of structural leg length inequality (LLI) is something of an elephant in the room that no one really wants to talk about. Well, we *are* going to talk about it, bring it stage center. Many cases of pelvic torsion are compensatory for structural LLI; in such cases, as discussed below, the prone or supine short leg shows up the side of anterior innominate rotation.

Changes in the lower extremity

Although it is not our intention to dwell on treatment of the lower extremity in this book, it is necessary to describe the kinetic chain that relates the lumbopelvis to the lower extremity.

> Physical findings on relaxed side pronated foot:
> - inferior hip
> - increased valgus angle, knee
> - internal rotation of tibia on foot
> - internal rotation of femur on tibia
> - internal rotation of pelvis on femur (external rotation of the hip)
> - lumbar lateral curvature

5. Theories of pelvic distortion

The clinical entity

The patient complains of chronic, diffuse low back pain with radiation to the buttocks. It occasionally disappears, but always returns, often after a fairly mild provocation, such as a game of tennis or an airplane flight. The pain is usually fairly mild, but can get fairly uncomfortable at times.

Physical examination will evidence no neurologic deficits. The principal findings will include areas of palpatory tenderness (myofascitis), muscle hypertonicity, postural deviations, usually mild orthopedic results, and some hypomobile joints. In a medical or physical therapy setting the patient will be diagnosed to suffer from "non-specific," "mechanical," "uncomplicated," or perhaps "postural" low back pain, or even more simply, "lumbar sprain/strain." The same patient in a chiropractic setting will be found to suffer from spinal/pelvic "subluxations." We have found it convenient to say that patients such as these have suffered an exacerbation of a "chronic postural sprain," or perhaps from "chronic postural subluxation." A related but more inclusive terminology would find the patient to present with a "postural distortion syndrome," a determinate full-body loss of postural neutrality in the sagittal and frontal planes.

In cases such as these, which are said to embrace up to 80-90% of low back pain patients, it is very difficult to determine which tissues are giving rise to the pain, let alone the cause(s) of the problem. Whatever the diagnosis, there is a growing body of literature that suggests that spinal manipulative therapy (SMT) is the treatment of choice, and the more so to the extent that the onset of the problem has been recent.

It is our purpose here to describe a broad-based clinical approach to cases such as these, broad-based in that it eclectically draws upon many the most cogent findings of many different chiropractic techniques and of allied health professionals. The approach herein described emphasizes postural indicators, not because they are necessarily more important than motion palpation findings, but because at this level of simplicity interexaminer reliability (and therefore cross-professional credibility) is increased.

It will be necessary to first discuss the joint architecture and kinematics of the lumbopelvic area. Following this we go on to describe the archetypical postural distortion syndrome which can be identified in this region, following which we present the clinical findings that are to be expected in this distortion model. Finally, the x-ray findings are described.

Although the chapter concludes with a description of the distortion cascade that relates to lumbopelvic distortion, with the implicit assumption that the lumbopelvic changes are primary in some ways, it would be possible to relax that assumption. Indeed, it may be possible to derive the lumbopelvic distortion from some other primary cause, ranging from upper cervical subluxation to pronation of the foot, at the opposite extreme. Starting from the lumbopelvis is more a matter of convenience in exposition than a theory, in the present work.,

The lumbopelvis

The pelvis is a kinematic chain involving six bones and six joints. The bones include the left and right innominate bones, the sacrum, the two femurs, and the coccyx. The six joints include the two hip joints, the two sacroiliac joints, the sacrococcygeal joint, and the symphysis pubis. The sacrum is lodged as a bridge in-between the two innominate bones, the three bones forming collectively the pelvic bowl. This structure constitutes a kinematic chain, insofar as movement at any one on these joints is necessarily associated with movement at various of the other joints.

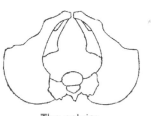

The pelvis:
3 bones, 3 joints

Movements at the hip joints

Three possible types of pelvic motion occur at the hip joints:

• A bilateral rocking of the entire pelvis may occur in the sagittal plane, around an axis through the hips. This axis is perpendicular to the sagittal plane. It is discussed below why there can be no opposed rotations of the two innominate bones about this axis; that is, one innominate cannot rotate clockwise while the other rotates counterclockwise, to any significant extent. Posterior rocking (hip extension) is limited by the tension developed in the very strong anterior iliofemoral ligament, an inverted Y-shaped ligament arising by its tail from the ASIS and attaching to the intertrochanteric line of the femur. Anterior rocking (hip flexion) is limited by the transversely oriented ischiofemoral ligament.

• A rotation of the entire pelvis around its center of gravity may occur in the transverse plane, around the Y (vertical) axis. This swings one hip anteriorward and the other posteriorward, perhaps to different degrees, in which case some unleveling of the femur heads might occur. One hip winds up becoming externally rotated and the other hip internally rotated.

• The entire pelvis may laterally shift to one side or another in the frontal plane, parallel to the X axis. If the hips are squarely planted above the ankles, with the knees and ankles in the neutral position, this motion *cannot unlevel the femur heads,* contrary to what one reads in some technique textbooks. Following sway, a line connecting the femur heads, and another connecting the feet, would form the top and bottom of a parallelogram. The hip on the side to which the pelvis sways is posturally adducted, whereas the other hip is posturally abducted.

Movements of the sacroiliac joints

At least two, and possibly three, motions take place at the sacroiliac joints. These can be best understood as simultaneous rotations around 3 axes. One of the reasons why descriptions of sacroiliac motions differ so much from book to book is that some authorities will speak of "translations" to get across the fact that the various axes of rotation are themselves in motion.

• Nutation and counternutation around the X axis

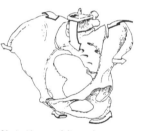

Nutation, obliquely seen, Lee's rendering of Kapandji's drawing.

The sacrum can bilaterally or unilaterally nutate (see figures to the right) which refers to an anterior-inferior rotation of its base relative to the ilium about an axis perpendicular to the sagittal plane, a motion which simultaneously swings the sacral apex posterior-superior. The anterior swing of the sacral base allows the iliac crests to draw closer together, insofar as the sacrum no longer splays them apart as much. This simultaneously means that the pubic bones will stretch apart slightly. The sacrum may also counter-nutate, which swings its base posterior-inferior and its apex anterior-superior. The sacrum acts like a wedge in forcing the iliac crests away from one another, which in turn causes an approximation at the symphysis pubis. Kapandji (The Physiology of the Joints, Volume III, p.64) limits the possible motion to 3 mm in either direction at the sacral base, and a total of 15 mm at the sacral apex. Nutation is limited by the tightening of the sacrotuberous and sacrospinous ligaments.

Sacral nutation and counternutation (from Kapandji).

Counternutation is limited by tension in the posterior and anterior sacroiliac ligaments. Not only can nutation occur unilaterally, but it may be accompanied by contralateral counternutation. A moment's reflection will establish that when this occurs, there must be associated rotation of the sacrum around a somewhat upright axis, as discussed in the next paragraph.

• Rotation around the "Y" axis (actually, an axis somewhat oblique to the Y axis)

The sacrum, according to Hildebrandt, can rotate between the two ilia about an axis perpendicular to its base an axis which therefore inclines anterior-superiorward in the sagittal plane. This rotation would move one aspect of the sacral base anterior and inferior with respect to the ipsilateral ilium, while the other aspect of its base would be brought posterior and superior.

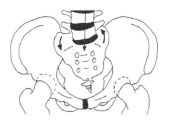

Sacral rotation around axis perpendicular to base, after Hildebrandt. Also shown, lateral sacral lateral flexion.

• Lateral flexion of the sacrum around the Z axis

The sacrum can laterally flex in the frontal plane relative to the ilia. Given the difficulty of establishing a universal frame of reference for this motion, one that would obtain universal agreement, it is hard to say what constitutes "left" or "right" lateral flexion of the sacrum. As we shall see, this creates little practical difficulty for us, since our only concern in this matter is to be able to clearly describe which way the apex points when pelvic torsion occurs, and this will not be difficult.

In reading descriptions of the sacroiliac motions, one notes that some authors (e.g., Weisel, Greenman) speak of linear translations. Actually, if one were to take into account that unilateral nutation and rotation in the plane of the sacral base take place simultaneously, the net effect is equivalent to such a translation. In other words, the instantaneous axis of rotation (IAR, discussed below) for sacral nutation is a moving target, in that its location changes as the sacral base rotates between the innominate bones. As a general rule, the movements of the sacrum are relatively small, although there is quite a spread in actual measurements going from one authority to another. As a pure coincidence, numbers like "2" and "3" keep coming up, whether the units are millimeters or degrees, per joint; and thus about 4-6 degree/millimeters of left-right difference in simultaneous, opposed movements.

Information now emerging from the physical therapy milieu (see Diane Lee's recent works and the text by her mentor, Vleeming), suggests that when the sacrum is nutated on the ilium, the sacroiliac joint is locked up, whereas it is unstable when the sacrum is counternutated. This would imply that in a pelvic torsional state, one would expect to find fixation (i.e., restriction) of the SI joint on the side of posterior innominate rotation, and a tendency towards misalignment on the anterior side (if that has occurred as well, it need not have). As is discussed below in another chapter, the Gonsteadian "posterior" sacrum might indeed represent this instability-bred subluxation of the sacrum relative to the ipsilateral innominate bone. Instability-*bred*, although it may wind up *restricted*, due to the splinting muscle spasm one would expect as the sacral base wedges apart the innominate bone in its posterior migration. Diane Lee addresses the paradox that misalignments born of instability wind up feeling restricted to an examiner, for which reason she recommends looking for left-right asymmetry of the quality of palpatory findings, rather than the more usual assessment of range of motion.

Movements at the symphysis pubis

The symphysis pubis is an amphiarthrodial joint which accommodates to torsional movements between the innominate bones, but normally is incapable of sheering motions (gliding movements), a type of motion that occurs only within diarthrodial, synovial joints. The symphysis pubis does exhibit some degree of compression during sacral counternutation and of distraction during sacral nutation, which is to say that it accommodates some types of innominate motion in the frontal plane: separation or approximation of the ASISs and/or PSISs. Vertical sheer within the symphysis pubis can only occur if there is trauma or ligamentous laxity as in pregnancy, or Ehlers-Danlos syndrome. (Kapandji, p.70). Unfortunately, various chiropractic theories of pelvic torsion, however unknowingly, require just such an unlikely vertical disruption of the symphysis pubis.

The actual amount of sheer that occurs at the symphysis, in relatively normal subjects (meaning, without gross ligamentous damage, who are not loaded up with relaxin during a pregnancy or immediately post-partum, who do have inflammatory arthritis, who do not have congenital diseases of hypermobility, like Ehlers-Danlos syndrome, etc.) is less than 2 millimeters. The joint has been studied by putting subjects in the straddle position, and/or in one-legged stance. Cadaveric studies have also been performed.

	Walheim (22)	Pitkin (23)	Greenman (24)	Death (25)
vertical translation	1.0 mm males 1.3 mm females		occurs during one-legged standing	0.81 ± 0.74 mm (0 to 2 mm)
sagittal plane rotation	0.3 to 0.8^0	5.5^0	occurs during gait	
frontal plane rotation	0.4^0			

The sacrococcygeal joint

The sacrococcygeal joint is an amphiarthrosis which performs essentially flexion and extension, occurring passively in defecation and in labor. It seems to play little part in all this, and need not concern us further in this analysis. (Logan said that the coccyx tended to point toward the side of the low sacrum, in his model of the "Basic Distortion.")

Theories of pelvic distortion

All descriptions of the "PI ilium" would agree that the posterior superior iliac spine (PSIS) has gone posterior and inferior - but with respect to what? Only occasionally do the clinicians seem to feel the need to clarify; much of the time we are forced to deduce what they have in mind from chance remarks here and there, and also on the basis of what they do clinically. Inconsistencies among authors and even in the work of an individual author abound.

In a state of perfect postural symmetry, the two innominate bones would be superimposed when the subject is viewed from the side. Failing this, a state of inter-innominate subluxation is assumed to exist. One can easily imagine various manners in which the innominate bones could lose their superimposition in the lateral view. Two main possibilities have been described: 1) one innominate might slip in a linear fashion with respect to the other one, a type of movement called "linear translation;" and 2) either or both innominates could rotate about some axis which is more or less perpendicular to the sagittal plane, resulting in pelvic torsion.

Linear translation misalignment of an innominate bone

Primarily osteopaths have described such "upslips" and "downslips" of the innominate bones, as might be described by the figure. A purely linear translation - whether inferior/superior or anterior/superior - is unlikely as a routine event, in that it would require a motion of the symphysis pubis which would be very unlikely for it, namely, a gliding or sheering motion. As described in the section on movements of the symphysis pubis, it is an amphiarthrosis which is capable of torsion and various bend-related deformations, but not normally of a linear translation, which remains an option only for a diarthrosis type of joint. Although some chiropractic drop-table practitioners describe some clinical situations in which the innominate may move posteriorly in a linear fashion, it is mostly the osteopathic profession that routinely describes such a misalignment.

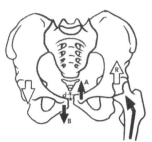

Standing on one leg puts shear force on symphysis, but normally the gap "d" does not open up. This constrains possible axes for pelvic torsion (Kapandji, p.71)

Rotational misalignment of the innominate bones

As the chiropractic readers know, most of us think that posterior innominate movement occurs in a rotatory manner. Let us consider a few examples of typical chiropractic rotational models of pelvic misalignment. Some would find the ilium PI with respect to the sacrum:

• "When the ilium becomes misaligned, it does so in relation to the sacrum, and the actual misalignment occurs in the sacroiliac articulation." (Herbst, The A-P Misalignment, p1).

Others would find, instead of or in addition to the statement above, that the ilium is PI with respect to the other ilium, and we can offer up several examples of this type of belief.

• "When an ilium misaligns in a PI direction, the length of the innominate involved increases on the A-P film...The larger of the two innominate measurements accompanies the PI ilium." (Herbst again, p.8-10).

• "The ilium goes posterior and inferior and the pivot point is the acetabulum" (Thompson, Thompson Technique Reference Manual, 1984, p.30).

• Hildebrandt's pelvic cleavage model (our favored theory, see below) is also of this ilk.

Whether explicitly or implicitly, these theories require the two innominate bones to be counter-rotated with respect to one another. They would be subluxated with respect to each other, to the sacrum, or to each other and the sacrum. Some (Thompson) would consider both ilia subluxated, whereas others (Gonstead) would consider subluxation of one the primary and of the other the compensation.

It should be possible to identify the axis around which the innominate bones accomplish their mutual counter-rotation. Clinicians have varied as to where this axis would be, but they have generally felt it to be either through the hip joint (Logan), the sacroiliac joint (Herbst, representing the Gonstead position, at least according to Hildebrandt), or somewhere in-between. Hildebrandt insists that innominate counter-rotation must place about an axis through the symphysis pubis. Let us see why he takes this position.

Pelvic torsion around the symphysis pubis

We may now describe the most common lumbopelvic postural distortion syndrome, subject to the anatomical parameters that have been described above.

We are going to tell the story from the point of view of the innominate bone, as if its subluxation were the precipitating event for the overall distortion. However, it will become apparent that the sacrum can not remain aloof from this process, as it would be torn asunder were the sacroiliac joints not to achieve endogenous compensation. In fact, the entire story could just as easily have been told from the point of view of the sacrum, as did Logan, or possibly even from that of the

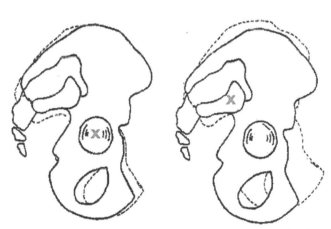

Pelvic torsion around hip axis would wreck the symphysis. Rotation around the SI would be worse. A hypothetical interinnominate rotation axis through the SI joint would be even worse than a hip pivot point. (Adapted from Hildebrandt)

lumbar spine. [It is recommended that the reader consult Hildebrandt's *Chiropractic Spinography* for further clarification of the discussion which follows.]

Chiropractors have emphasized the possibility of opposed, mutual rotations of the innominate bones. In order to visualize the mechanism of pelvic torsion

(Hildebrandt likes to call it torsion), the reader need only imagine twisting a model of the pelvic girdle, each hand gripping one of the iliac crests and "wringing" it in opposite directions as if it were a wet bath towel. It would be better yet if the reader were to actually perform this experiment on a model of the pelvis; it would be noted that little differences in the way the twisting is executed change the degree to which mechanical stress is exerted on the sacroiliac joints and the symphysis pubis. It's all a question of what is chosen to be the pivot point for the twisting motion, its axis of rotation. It can be readily seen that any appreciably posterior location of this axis would tend to dislocate the symphysis pubis. If, for example, the axis were an axle running through the two femur heads (as many chiropractors seem to think it is), then twisting about this axis would cause a significant elevation of the pubic bone on the PI side, and a relative descent of the pubic bone on the other side. For the reasons stated above this appears unlikely to occur.

The situation would be significantly worse were the axis to run through the sacroiliac joints, as some chiropractors would have it. Indeed, to get .5" of PSIS unleveling, the pelvis would have to pay the price of approximately 1.5" of symphysis pubis dislocation.

It turns out that the only location of the axis that does not require the symphysis to accommodate in an impossible manner is through the symphysis pubis itself (see 3 figures below, featuring a symphysis axis of rotation. This of course exerts a mechanical stress upon the sacroiliac joints; however, the diarthrodial nature of these joints, as described in the section above on the motion of the sacroiliac joints, permits them to accommodate for the pelvic torsion. Later in this text, in the chapter on the roentgenometrics of the pelvis, some calculations are presented for how much PSIS unleveling may result from SI motions. It turns out that the asymmetries that clinicians report turn out to be quite plausible in most cases.

Pelvic cleavage and the PI ilium

Pelvic cleavage is more or less equivalent to the conventional chiropractic listing of "PI ilium." This latter nomenclature is inadequate, insofar as the innominate bone is constrained to swing medially as well when it subluxates in a posteroinferior direction. This is owing to the fact that the sacroiliac joints possess an oblique orientation, one in which they converge posteriorly. The proper listing would therefore have to be "PI-medial" ilium." (Classic chiropractic listing terminology would refer to this an a "PI-IN ilium.") As a corollary, it is difficult to imagine how, in the absence of serious ligamentous damage or laxity, an ilium could subluxate posteroinferior and lateral ("PI-EX"). Analogously, the innominate is constrained to move laterally when its PSIS moves anterosuperiorly. These points should become more clear as the analysis develops, especially in the section on sacral accommodation to pelvic cleavage.

Hildebrandt, believing himself to have discovered that the axis for interinnominate torsion must pass through the symphysis, humbly calls this the Hildebrandt theory. However, this has been described at least since the seminal Pitkin and Pheasant paper of 1936, and has more recently been confirmed by a number of anatomical studies.

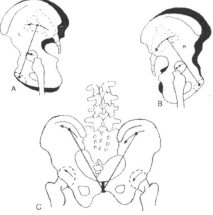

Pelvic torsion as portrayed by Hildebrandt. A=anterior rotation, B=posterior rotation, C=torsion as seen in frontal plane.

Sacral accommodation

Even though we have so far saved the symphysis pubis, we have now posed a grave danger to the sacrum, which must constitute a bridge connecting the left and right ilia, which are no longer in the same position in the sagittal plane. The sacrum would indeed be forced to sheer were it not for its ability to offset the cleavage of the two ilia by two types of motion: it can nod its base forward in the sagittal plane, and it can rotate between the two ilia in the plane which is defined by its base.

If the left innominate bone were to rock posterior and inferior, the left sacroiliac joint moves in this same direction. The sacroiliac ligaments are stretched by this motion, which means that although the sacrum must "go with the ilium," it does so incompletely. If the PSIS were to translate posteriorly say 6 mm, then the sacroiliac ligament may stretch by some 2 mm so that the left sacral base translates by only 4 mm posterior. (These numbers are for the purpose of illustration only, and not to be accepted as accurate.) This means that the sacrum is now positioned 2 mm *anterior to the same side innominate bone*, even though both the left innominate and sacrum *are posterior to the other side of the pelvis.* [Although no one ever notices this, the sacrum also incompletely follows the innominate bone inferiorly, so it is left slightly superior with respect to the innominate bone, although inferior to the other side of the sacral base.] We will see the

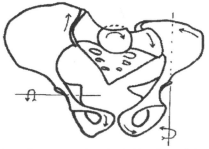

Sacral gyroscopic adaptation to pelvic cleavage: nutation/counternutation, base rotation, lateral flexion. From Grieve.

importance of these distinctions when we get to the section on chiropractic listings, where we attempt to establish an anatomically correct table of conversions for the different techniques. To get ahead of the story, although all chiropractor wind up agreeing that the sacral base is inferior on one side, some will find it simultaneously anterior (the AI sacrum) whereas others will find it posterior (the posterior-inferior sacrum.) This discrepancy will have to be resolved.

We have already seen that the innominate bone rocks posteriormedial as well. Again, the sacroiliac ligaments stretch a bit, so that the sacrum travels medial with it, but incompletely. This amounts to saying that the sacrum rotates its body away from the posterior-inferior-medial innominate bone. For example, in the case of a left PI ilium, the sacral body in effect turns to the right, relative to the innominate bone (although not necessarily in absolute terms.)

The sacrum in fact is capable of functioning like a gyroscope between the ilia, instantly compensating for this pelvic cleavage. It compensates for the posteroinferior motion of the innominate bone by unilaterally nutating on the same side; it compensates for the medial aspect of the innominate's swing by rotating the sacral body contralaterally, toward the other innominate bone. It turns in this opposed direction around an axis which is erected perpendicular to its base. It also laterally flexes. All of these sacral motions are depicted in the figure These accommodations are not necessarily affected by means of muscular contraction, insofar as they are automatic consequences of the sacroiliac joint architecture and the inherent ability of the sacroiliac ligament to stretch.

Left sacral base anterior to ipsilateral innominate, and posterior to right sacral base.

The figure portrays how the sacrum can be regarded as simultaneously "posterior" and "anterior" at the same time in this distortion; posterior in relationship to the contralateral side of the sacrum, anterior in relationship to the ipsilateral innominate bone. Might this reconcile the Logan "anterior-inferior" sacrum with the Gonstead "posterior-inferior" sacrum? Almost: it would take a redefinition of the posterior-inferior sacrum, so that "posterior" is interpreted in relation to the other side of the sacrum, not the innominate bone.

The distortion cascade

Pelvic cleavage represents a perturbation of the body's static equilibrium position, a disturbance of its condition of postural neutrality. The body's attempt to homeostatically govern this posture will be reflected in other regions departing from their posturally neutral position as well, in order to accommodate and compensate for the pelvic cleavage. We are forced to assume that the disturbance is at least partially damped, in that the effects of the disruption recede the greater the distance from the pelvis. For example, one would expect the fifth lumbar to be more affected by the sacral inferiority than the ninth thoracic. This assumed damping is an intrinsic component of the postural homeostatic mechanism. Separate units are devoted to some of these regional consequences of the pelvic cleavage, but they should be listed in this section in order that we get a glimpse of the big picture effect now that we have waded through the details of the pelvic mechanism.

Lumbar spine

The fifth lumbar is perched precariously on top of a sacroiliac joint which has slid posterior and inferior. We will need to see how it responds, and how this effects the other lumbar vertebra both in the frontal and sagittal planes. The lumbar spine attempts to maintain its perpendicular relationship to the pelvic girdle. Failures to compensate appropriately for unleveling of the pelvis, whether due to pelvic torsion or anatomical leg length inequality, tend to occur at the L4-5 articulation.

Thoracic spine

Likewise, the thoracic spine will be forced to accommodate itself to positional alterations within the lumbopelvic area. The body quite naturally must maintain balance; any alteration in lumbopelvic weight distribution must be offset in the thoracic (and to a lesser extent cervical) spine, in order that the body not keel over either laterally, backward, or forward. Events in the thoracic spine are very much constrained and delimited by the stabilizing presence of the rib cage.

The cervical spine and cranium

In turn, the craniocervical spine must adjust to altered thoracolumbopelvic position. If the rib cage can be said to define thoracic possibilities, in the same manner the vital importance of the neural structures that are lodged within the cervical spine and the cranium will very much delimit and constrain the accommodation responses that occur in this region. For example, the proper functioning of stereoscopic vision requires that the eyes be held level, which is probably the most stringent initial condition for the determination of local craniocervical equilibrium.

The shoulder girdle

Given that the cervicothoracic spine is in a state of accommodation for lumbopelvic events, the shoulder girdle in turn must accommodate itself to cervicothoracic events. Let us recall that the arms are evolutionarily designed for brachiation, and that the shoulder girdle is therefore rather loosely attached to the axial skeleton. Its positional orientation is governed more by the overall status of muscular contractions than it is by the intrinsic joint architecture of its internal joints (sternoclavicular, glenohumeral, acromioclavicular, and the scapulothoracic articulation). The shoulder girdle (teleologically speaking) "wants" to remain perpendicular to the spine, just as the lumbar spine in its accommodation to pelvic cleavage would like to remain reasonably perpendicular to the pelvic girdle.

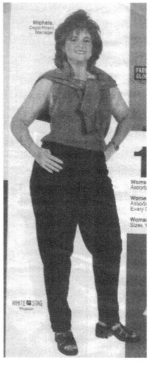

The lower extremities

The most interesting consequence of pelvic cleavage, as far as the leg is concerned, is what Hildebrandt refers to as the "physiological lengthening" of the femur. In other words, the posteroinferiomedial swing of the innominate bone about a symphysis pubis pivot necessarily swings the femur head as well inferiorly. We will have to see how and why the foot is not propelled in this manner through the floor. It should be noted that in this model the acetabulum is not elevated by the innominate rotation, the hypothetical (and incorrect) mechanism by which almost all clinicians have explained the finding of a physiological short leg. An entire unit is devoted to the consequences of the pelvic cleavage model for the interpretation of physiological leg length inequality. (Don't worry, the prone short leg is still on the PI side!)

The knee and ankle joints will have to accommodate for alterations in the hip position, both in terms of its elevation and position in the sagittal plane. Let us take note of the fact that the pelvic cleavage has carried the left innominate bone posterior, and the right innominate bone anterior: this means that entire pelvis is rotated counterclockwise around the Y axis of the body. (For some individuals it is counterintuitive that turning to the left represents clockwise rotation around the Y axis of the body.) A person cannot effectively confront three dimensions while initiating ambulation from a pelvis that is not facing forward. Although the entire body in a sense will participate in the attempt to solve this problem, the biomechanical stress seems to be maximized in the very complicated and therefore vulnerable ankle and knee joints. Alterations in the knee Q-angle and foot pronation are part and parcel of this model and will have to be carefully examined.

6. Lumbar adaptation to pelvic distortion

Although there are chapters below that address the lumbar spine in a general way, we herein discuss typical lumbar response patterns to pelvic torsion. These vary from the well-behaved "Basic Distortion" of Hugh Logan, in which L5 forms a well-behaved rotatory curvature, convex on the side of posterior innominate rotation, to poorly behaved distortions in which the curvature is excessive, non-existent, or even reversed. Sometimes the curvature "does the right thing," but the spinous processes remain on the midline or even deviate toward the convexity, forming a "simple" scoliosis.

The rotation and tipping of L5

Previously, we determined that the sacral base on the PI-medial side of innominate cleavage had gone inferior with respect to the other side of the sacrum. What about the fifth lumbar? What will it do, faced with this inferiority of its base of support?

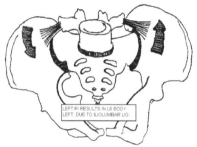

Note role of iliolumbar ligaments.

Although the position of L5 is not completely determinate, it is likely that it will sag on the side of its low base of support. Furthermore, it is likely that its body will rotate to the this same side, for at least two reasons. First, given that the weight of the body is transmitted to the legs primarily through the bodies of the vertebra, rather than through its facets, the law of gravity requires L5 to turn its body to the left. What's more, the iliolumbar ligament, approximating the transverse process to iliac crest, will necessarily turn the body of L5 to the low sacrum side as the ilium itself rotates posteriorly on the this same side. Quite naturally, the other iliolumbar ligament will pull the contralateral transverse process of L5 anteriorward as the pelvis cleaves anteriorward on other side of the body.

The figure (from Friberg[1]) demonstrates how that L5 body rotation looks from above. Notice that the patient turns his entire pelvis on the Y axis so that the posteriorly rotated innominate bone is carried anteriorly. Logan had detected this effect many years ago, and used the listing left or right "anterior pelvis" to describe such Y axis rotation of the pelvis anteriorly on the PI side. Please do do

---

[1] Friberg O. Leg length inequality and low back pain. Clinical Biomechanics 1987;2:211-219.

confuse the "AS" listing, which has to do with sagittal plane rotations, with the "anterior pelvis, which has to do with Y axis rotation.

Lateral flexion of the spine as a pure motion does not occur, it is always accompanied by an element of twisting. In a normal lordotic lumbar spine, the vertebral bodies rotate away from the side of lateral bending, so that the spinous processes rotate toward the concavity created by the bend. In effect, the subject turns away from the side of desired lateral flexion and then extends toward it, putting his or her spine into hyperlordosis. The implications for spinal adjusting are developed later in this text, in the chapter on the vectored lumbothoracic adjustment (chapter 15).

The lower lumbar spine in the figure below forms a left convexity, the result of L5 being laterally tipped to the left. The need to maintain body balance dictates that either the upper lumbar spine or perhaps the lower thoracic spine will form a compensate right convexity, or right lateral curvature. The resultant s-shaped thoracolumbar spinal configuration tends to maintain the body's center of gravity over the middle of the sacral base.

The helical component of the lumbar distortion

Continuing up the spine, L4 is pulled posterior on the left by L5, but incompletely. Indeed, the spinous of L4 is to the right of the midline, although to the left of that of L5. Likewise for L3: its spinous is to the right of the midline, but to the left of the spinous of L4. A moment's reflection will establish the following: each segment in the lumbopelvic kinematic chain remains anterior on the left with respect to the segment below, and posterior on the left with respect to the one above. For further clarification of this spiral structure of the spine, the reader is referred to

(Data from Friberg)	
Segment	Mean torsion
L1-L2	0.79
L2-L3	0.97
L3-L4	1.06
L4-L5	1.35
L5-S1	-5.39

Johnston's article.[2] He was able to predict, using a wooden model, what Friberg demonstrated through his own careful x-ray study. The table shows the intersegmental rotations, in degrees, as measured by Friberg.

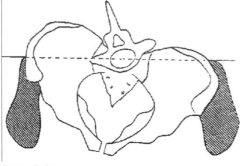

From Friberg.

The net effect of all this is that there is a helical component to the distortion pattern of the lumbar spine, a twist around the y-axis of the body. Friberg has calculated the mean intersegmental rotations for a large group of individuals presenting with low back pain. He did not consider the possibility of sacroiliac participation in the helix. What he calls "L5-S1" rotation is in fact, judging from the methodology he describes, L5-pelvis rotation, which includes a two-joint complex: the SI and L/S joints. This probably explains why he gets such a large value here, compared with the other lumbar intersegmental rotations.

We will see how the cervico-thoracic spine and head compensates for this twisting of the lower part in another section of the text. Obviously, there must be an opposite twisting somewhere above the lumbopelvis in order that the eyes gaze directly forward. This point has been estimated to be in the mid to lower thoracic spine.

Janse-Illi L5-S1 torsional effect

Drs. Janse and Illi described a mechanism by which lumbosacral torsion could develop: the sacrum subluxates anteriorly with respect to the innominate bone which is relatively posterior; the transverse process of the fifth lumbar vertebra is tethered to the iliac crest by virtue of the iliolumbar ligament, which therefore drags the fifth lumbar body posterior as well. The net result of these effects would be that the sacral base is anteriorly subluxated with respect to both the innominate bone and

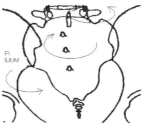

Left PI ilium and L5 body rotate clockwise on Y axis, while sacrum rotates counterclockwise.

the fifth lumbar. It might be the case that the lumbosacral joint, which many physical anthropologists consider quite exposed by the development of the bipedal posture and gait, may have evolved this locking mechanism to protect the lumbosacral disk from excessive rotation when the subject is standing on an

---

[2] Johnston LC. The paradox of the functional spine. Journal of the Canadian Chiropractic Association 1966(June-July):7-10.

unlevel surface. This is a typical circumstance in which the innominate bones cleave.

Compensatory torsion of the lower extremity

We will examine in another passage of the text we describe how it is that the upper part of the body compensates for this twisting that occurs in the lumbopelvic kinematic chain. There is, however, one component of compensation that is achieved by the lower part of the body that we should address right now.

When one innominate bone rotates posteriorly on the left, and the other anteriorly on the right, the pelvic bowl would wind up facing somewhat to the left were it not for yet another compensatory postural change. The entire pelvis rotates around the y axis of the body, turning to the right (counterclockwise). With the feet planted on the ground, this creates in effect external rotation of the left hip, and medial rotation of the left tibia on the foot, pronating the foot. Dr. Hugh Logan called the net result of this compensatory pattern a "left anterior pelvis," not to be confused with a left anterior-superior ilium. The anterior pelvis listing refers to y-axis rotation, whereas the anterior-superior ilium refers to rotation around the x-axis.

Overall assessment of the lumbar spine and pelvis

What follows simply serves as an introduction to a more comprehensive discussion of patient evaluation in a subsequent chapter. It is best to get behind the standing patient to determine whether or not there appears to be a significant degree of pelvic torsion. This becomes apparent not only through direct inspection and palpation of the pelvis, but also from evaluation of the lower extremities.

Imagine a pelvis which (1) appears level, which (2) is not rotated much on the Y axis, which (3) sits on top of lower extremities that are symmetric in terms of the arches of the feet, the Q-angles of the knee, and the degree of hip rotation. Obviously, such a pelvis probably does not manifest intrapelvic torsion. By comparison, a pelvis which does show all or some of these parameters probably is in a torsional state.

If the pelvis is symmetric, and yet the lumbar spine exhibits obvious lateral curvature, more often than not there is a segmental lesion of L4-5. Barge called this a "disk block subluxation," that gave rise to the condition "tortipelvis." L5 is quite tightly tethered to the innominate bones by the iliolumbar ligaments, which prevent the disc block from occurring at the L5-S1 articulation. The disc block subluxation may, however, show up more cephalad in the lumbar spine, the listing in Gonstead language being a PRS or PLS.

Actually, there are a number of lumbopelvic patterns, which have become known to us as Lovett relationships, after the influential early 20th century authority on scoliosis. He himself did not, to our knowledge, attach his name to any of the patterns, reprinted here as appendix 1.

In the sagittal plane, it is common to find hyperextension of the lumbosacral joint, of L4/5, or of both. This postural fault should be distinguished from sway-back (an anterior translation of the entire pelvis) and from true hyperlordosis (global participation of the lumbar vertebra in exaggerated lordosis, e.g., L2-S1. True hyperlordosis of the lumbar spine is usually seen in relatively older people, where it may accompany degenerative spondylolistheses. It is also seen among very deconditioned, and very obese people.

Summary of components of pelvic torsion

At this point it might be useful to summarize some of the grand contours of the argument. Many different authorities both in and out of chiropractic have described a model similar to this one. It bears most resemblance to Logan's "Basic Distortion" which itself is patterned after the work of Carver and of Lovett. (In relationship to the latter, whose book *Lateral Curvature of the Spine and Round Shoulders* gave rise to the so-called "Lovett system of scoliosis classification," this model would be called a "Lovett positive.")

The lumbar spine goes into a rotatory scoliosis on the side of the low sacrum, which occurs on the side of the posterior innominate bone. It might be useful to recapitulate the key events in this distortion as if there were a direct, linear causal relationship among them, even though in reality the findings present as a syndrome in which all the separate components mutually and simultaneously co-determine each other. In the chapter on the clinical findings, we will more linearly describe various clinical signs of this PI ilium postural distortion syndrome.

• Allow the left innominate to rotate posteriorly and the right innominate to rotate relatively anteriorly about a symphysis pubis axis.

• The left sacroiliac joint experiences a posterior-inferior-medial subluxation in relation to the other sacroiliac joint.

• The left aspect of the sacral base is lowered with the left innominate bone, to which it is tightly articulated.

• The sacral base on the left winds up unilaterally nutated around the x-axis, because it is left somewhat anterior to the posteriorly rotated left innominate bone. In other words, the left sacroiliac ligament is stretched by the posterior innominate rotation: the sacral base goes with the innominate, but incompletely.

• In addition to nutating around the x-axis, the sacrum has another way of winding up anterior on the left: it rotates around the "y-axis" (actually, an axis perpendicular to the sacral base, somewhat oblique to the actual y-axis). As the left posterior-inferior-medial ilium moves medially, the sacrum travels with it, but incompletely. In effect the sacral base rotates counterclockwise between the ilia (anteriorly on the left in relation to the left innominate bone).

• The sacrum laterally flexes, such that its apex points towards the right, since its base has gone inferiorward on the left. This amounts to rotation about the z-axis.

• The fifth lumbar body both rotates clockwise with the left innominate bone, tethered by the iliolumbar ligaments, and sags inferiorly on the left, as its base of support, the sacral base, moves inferiorly as well.

• The lumbar spine assumes a helical distortion, a rotatory scoliosis in which each vertebra is turned counterclockwise on the y-axis in relation to the one below, even though at least the lower segments will have their spinous processes to the right of the midline of the body.

• The left hip is externally rotated, creating left foot flare.

• The left tibia, in an effort to maintain a forward facing, winds up medially rotated in relation to the flared foot, thus pronating it.

• The left femur is in turn medially rotated with respect to the left tibia, accounting for an increase in the knee's Q-angle, or a condition of genu valgum.

• The left knee and hip flex slightly.

Sagittal plane lumbar adaptations

It stands to reason that the inclination of the pelvis will impact on the sagittal plane configuration of the lumbar spine. The steeper the pelvic tilt angle, the more

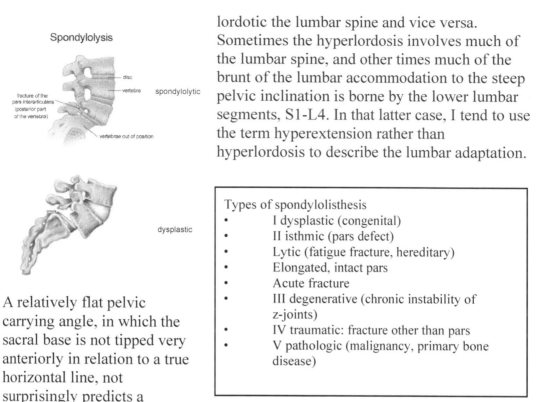

Spondylolysis

disc
vertebra — spondylolytic
fracture of the
pars interarticularis
(posterior part
of the vertebra)
vertebrae out of position

dysplastic

lordotic the lumbar spine and vice versa. Sometimes the hyperlordosis involves much of the lumbar spine, and other times much of the brunt of the lumbar accommodation to the steep pelvic inclination is borne by the lower lumbar segments, S1-L4. In that latter case, I tend to use the term hyperextension rather than hyperlordosis to describe the lumbar adaptation.

Types of spondylolisthesis
- I dysplastic (congenital)
- II isthmic (pars defect)
- Lytic (fatigue fracture, hereditary)
- Elongated, intact pars
- Acute fracture
- III degenerative (chronic instability of z-joints)
- IV traumatic: fracture other than pars
- V pathologic (malignancy, primary bone disease)

A relatively flat pelvic carrying angle, in which the sacral base is not tipped very anteriorly in relation to a true horizontal line, not surprisingly predicts a relatively diminished lumbar lordosis. It is not uncommon to witness a very straight lumbar spine perched upon a small lordosis spanning the lower 2-3 segments alone.

Exaggerated lumbar lordosis shifts weight onto the posterior zygapophysis, thus increasing the likelihood of facet syndrome; whereas a diminished lumbar lordosis shifts body weight toward the anterior zygapophysis, increasing the pounds per square inch on the intervertebral disc, thus elevating the risk of disc disease (at least in the long run).

Hyperlordosis increases the risk of spondylolisthesis, in which the body of L5 literally slides downhill on the steeply inclined surface of the sacral base. There are many types of spondylolisthesis, as can b be seen in the table. The figure shows two of the types, spondylolytic and dysplastic spondylolisthesis. Both are amenable to adjustive proceedures, as are discussed later in the book.

It should be pointed out that the finding of a spondylolisthesis on an x-ray is always a dramatic event, often unsuspected. Given the power of images, it is understandable how this often amounts to a "eureka moment," where both the doctor and patient share an understanding that the true cause of the symptoms have been found. However, I believe this is generally premature. Although images are compelling, the hyperlordosis that serves as a risk factor for spondylolisthesis may be the primary cause of the low back pain, rather than the spondylolisthesis itself. Fortunately, the preferred corrective procedure discussed later in the book, a side-posture technique developed from the Pettibon system, would be expected to address lumbar hyperlordosis as much as it would spondylolisthesis per se. Thus, clinical benefit would be expected, irrespective as to whether the spondylolisthesis is the primary cause or rather simply associated with the underlying cause, hyperlordosis.

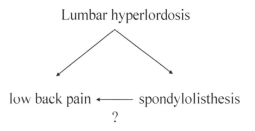

Appendix: Lovett classification of scolioses

The Lovett concept of curvature evaluation is an early day method of classifying lumbar spine scolioses in accordance with their functional/structural characteristics and clinical significance. Six types have been described.

A. <u>Lovett Positive</u>
The vertebral bodies rotate compensatorily toward the side of the scoliosis convexity, which is on the low side of a deviated sacral base. The angle of the vertebral plane at both ends of the scoliosis is in conformity with that of the sacrum. This type is a competently developed compensation to an unleveling of the sacral base and is generally asymptomatic.

B. <u>Lovett Static</u>
Convexity of scoliotic deviation is toward the low side of an unleveled sacral base, but without body rotation. This type is usually symptomatic and suggests moderate spasm of the psoas and multifidous muscles on the side of scoliotic convexity.

C. <u>Lovett Negative</u>
There is a scoliotic deviation to the low side of an unleveled sacral base, but vertebral body rotation is toward the side of scoliotic concavity. This type tends to be acutely symptomatic and suggests severe spasm of psoas and multifidous muscles on the convex side of the scoliosis.

D. <u>Lovett Failure</u>
The sacrum is deviated low on one side or the other but the lumbar spine remains straight--without scoliotic deviation or compensations. This situation suggests bilateral psoas and multifidous muscle spasm and is said to be frequently associated with disk disorder.

E. <u>Lovett Excess</u>
There is a scoliotic deviation with the vertebral bodies rotated toward the side of a low sacral base, but the degree of vertebral body deviation and scoliotic deviation are in excess to that which would be suggested by the degree of sacral base lowering. This type suggests: (a) an undue spasm of the psoas and multifidous muscles on the high side of the sacral base, (b) a possible wedging of the L5 vertebra on the low side of sacral deviation and/or (c) a loosening of the disk and ligamentous restraining structures.

F. <u>Lovett Reverse</u>
There is a scoliotic deviation to the high side of the sacral base due to marked wedging of L4 or L5, or severe spasm of the psoas and multifidous muscles on the low side of the sacral base. Marked hypoplasia of the lumbosacral facets may also be suspect on the side of the high sacral base and side of atypical scoliotic convexity.

(adapted from Erhardt)

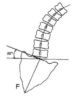

7. Examining and assessing the lumbopelvis

This chapter, after briefly reviewing the kinematics of the lumbar spine, deals with a few general issues relative to manual medicine. It eventually describes a clinical protocol for evaluating the lumbopelvic area.

Movements of the lumbar spine

The range of motion for flexion-extension gradually increases as we descend in the lumbar spine, starting at 12 degrees between L1 and L2, and attaining its maximum of 20 degrees at the lumbosacral joint, especially when the lumbosacral facets exhibit a sagittal facing. Each of the motor units shows about the same amount of lateral flexion, some 6 degrees, except for the lumbosacral joint which exhibits only half as much, some 3 degrees. Axial rotation is very limited, amounting to about 2 degrees per segment on the average but increasing up to 5 degrees in the lumbosacral joint. Since injuries to the disc occur usually under loads in which lateral flexion is combined with torsion, the marked limitation of lateral flexion in the lumbosacral joint appears to reduce the danger of rotational injury.

When a subject attempts a lateral bend with the thoracolumbar spine in the forward flexed position, the lumbar bodies turn toward the side of the lateral bend; whereas when a subject attempts a lateral bend with the spine extended, the opposite occurs, the vertebral bodies rotating away from the side of bend. Since the subject normally carries the lumbar spine in extension, the spinous processes therefore generally move toward the concavity of the lateral curve. This effect is probably exaggerated by the manner in which motion palpation is usually performed, where the subject is tested while sitting on a bar-type stool with the spine held in hyperlordosis.

Investigators have looked at both the quantitative and qualitative characteristics of lumbar coupling patterns, and especially their relationship to patient symptoms.[1] They found that "aberrant" coupling - that is, rotation of the spinous process toward the convex side - was so common that it might be as normal as "normal coupling," with rotation of the spinous process toward the concave side.

---

[1] Haas M, Peterson D. A roentgenological evaluation of the relationship between segmental motion and malalignment in lateral bending. Journal of Manipulative and Physiological Therapeutics 1991;15(6):350-360.

No correlation was detected between patient symptoms and either the type of quantity of lumbar segmental or regional motion.

Lumbar static and dynamic assessment

Hypomobility and hypermobility

The first point to be made is that what is commonly called "motion palpation" includes procedures that primarily assess joint *excursion*; and others that address end-range joint *stiffness*, or access to the paraphysiological joint space. Some of the dynamic assessment procedures, like the Gillet test, are more excursion-related, and others, like Lee's procedure for the assessing SI movement, assess the quality of end-range movements.

Turning to the sacroiliac joints, the Gillet step test is well-known. Versions of it are used in chiropractic, osteopathy, physical therapy, and physiatry. There are suggestions in the literature that the procedure entertains an acceptable degree of inter-rater reliability. (There are also suggestions it does not, especially a study in which the investigators threw a couple of ankylosing spondylitis subjects into the mix, who lacked discernable SI joints; the blinded investigators could not identify even them as restricted [2].) In the simplest variation on the theme, the examiner places one thumb on the PSIS, and the other on S2. The patient, facing the wall and stabilizing him or herself with his outstretched hands, is asked to raise the knee on his tested side toward his chest. If the ipsilateral SI joint is mobile, the thumb on the PSIS will drop relative to the other thumb on S2, indicating normal nutation of the sacrum on the posteriorly rotating innominate bone. The fluid motion test on the prone patient, described in the *Palmer Chiropractic College Adjusting Manual*, is also said to test for sacroiliac mobility. Physiotherapist Diane Lee favors placing the fingers of one hand on the sacral base, and the PSIS of the supine patient, while stressing the SI joint through cephalad pressure on the patient's ipsilateral lower extremity (I have not yet tried this procedure).

As for the lumbar facetal joints, I have always found motion palpation for excursion extremely difficult, for all regions of the spine, but have more conviction in procedures to identify end-range stiffness. This involves applying firm pressure using the same finger to alternate between the left and right sides of the spine, on the transverse processes, looking for differences in stiffness. When a stiff (hypomobile) joint is identified, the patient will generally confirm the

---

1. Mior SA, McGregor M, Schut B. The role of experience in clinical accuracy. J Manipulative Physiol Ther 1990;13(2):68-71.

tenderness. This same procedure applies, not surprisingly to the thoracic spine, and I use a similar supine procedure for the cervical spine.

My favored approach to assessing the dynamic properties of the lumbar spine is to have the patient laterally flex to each side, noting the contours of the spinous processes as this action is carried out. Normally, a smooth curve should be traced out, with neither "kinks" (local hypermobile discontinuities) nor "flattened" (non-participating hypomobile segments) areas. Certainly, there should never be a local convexity on the side to which the spine is laterally bending, which, if present, would indicate a structural, primary lateral curvature of the spine. *De facto*, I examine the lumbar and thoracic spines together in this regard. Since I discuss this procedure in some detail in the thoracic spine chapter, I would ask the reader to consult this chapter for clarification of this very simple and useful assessment vehicle.

Motion palpation studies have tended not to show very good reliability in the lumbar spine. In our own end-feel study, we were not able to achieve a high level of concordance, unlike our results in the thoracic spine, by changing the methodology in two ways: first, using continuous analysis, amenable to ICC and rather the Kappa statistic; and second, using confidence calls.

It is also useful to press P to A on each of the lumbar joints of the prone patient, as has already been described above in one of the introductory chapters, looking for differences in access to the paraphysiological joint space, left vs. right. Where excursion is difficult to determine, one can at least assess asymmetry in the quality of movement. One would also note any soft tissue textural changes, since spinal dysfunction is often associated with a thickening of the overlying soft tissue, that can be detected with a skin rolling maneuver, discussed more in the chapter on the thoracic spine below.

Lumbothoracic bending patterns

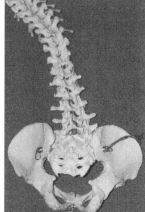

The doctor takes the patient to the passive end range of lateral flexion, left and right, examining for lumbothoracic spinal areas which do not participate in lateral flexion or which participate excessively. It is typical that at the base of a region that is restricted in lateral flexion to a given side there is a segment which is hypermobile in that same direction. Later, when we turn towards adjusting strategies for findings such as these, we will make the point that a line of drive that would worsen the situation of the hypermobile segment is to be eschewed, and lines of drives (and setups)

Lumbar spine shows region that does not participate in left lateral flexion that tend to reduce the flexion restriction are desirable.

Postural assessment

When we examine the standing patient, one of the most pertinent data points is whether the pelvis is level or not. That determines to a large extent the behavior of the lumbothoracic spine, given that 80% of spinal curvatures present as a lumbar convexity on the side of an inferior base of support, usually with an opposing thoracic curvature. It is important to realize that the standing PSIS and sacral base heights are the additive result of many contributory factors: anatomic LLI, pelvic cleavage, pronation (considered a component of anatomic LLI by some, and a functional derangement by others), different valgus angles at the knee, and asymmetric hip and/or knee flexion.

Among these various factors, assuming some that the examiner does not allow the subject to assume a *relaxed stance* posture, we need not worry about hip or knee flexion, nor do we suspect that typical Q angle differences would have much of a quantitative impact. We believe pronation to be a dependent variable, which reflects the additive impact of torsion (posterior innominate rotation lowers the sacral base, while anterior rotation elevates it) and anatomic LLI, which have more the character of independent variables. Anatomic LLI may add to this effect, neutralize it, or even reverse it. We must keep these relationships in mind as we go through the significance of many of the examination parameters that are discussed in this chapter.

Although our emphasis is on model building, we must also keep in mind that there are several clinical circumstances that tend to reduce the predictive power of models. Some of these constitute exceptions that prove the proverbial rule, and others prove a more general rule, to the effect "anything can happen." Here are some of these circumstances:

• Congenital anomalies such as spatulation of L5 or transitional lumbosacral segment, sacral asymmetry, spina bifida occulta, L5 hemivertebra or wedged shape, facetal tropism, etc.
• Weak ligaments: post-traumatic, associated with poor nutrition or old age, or related to pregnancy and the post-partum state. This may also result in any of the various listheses.
• Atypical or primary muscle spasm: that is, acute sprain/strain, as opposed to chronic postural sprain/strain.
• Intervertebral disc syndrome: a special case of spasm, usually presenting with antalgic lean.
• Inflammatory arthritis, e.g. osteitis condensans.

We are now in a position to identify some of the clinical signs of pelvic postural distortion, including torsion. No torsional patient will present with a completely consistent pattern, and yet if one notes how much of the evidence stacks up on the right and how much on the left, one will have a fairly well-based clinical impression as to the patient's distortion pattern. No such procedure is infallible. Patients who present with inconsistent patterns may have innominate cleavage with a failure of the lumbar spine to compensate, or perhaps a lumbar lateral curvature without evidence of pelvic torsion. These individuals simply do not present with a simple torsion syndrome. The author, who admits to being somewhat obsessed with pelvic torsion, apologizes in advance for having geared so much of the discussion that follows towards this unique clinical entity, as though it were the universal diagnosis of low back patients. It is not.

Carriage of innominate bone

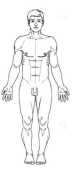

In the standing position, one iliac crest may be visualized and palpated to be inferior to the contralateral iliac crest. Again, this may result from pelvic torsion, anatomic LLI, or any combination thereof. In the appendix below on actual and projected innominate vertical length, some calculations are presented which indicate that for any given displacement of the iliac crests due to pelvic torsion, there will about twice as much discrepancy of the PSISs. This is because when the innominate bone rotates posteriorly around a symphysis axis, the high point of the crest moves relatively posterior, whereas the PSIS moves relatively inferior. Although both PSIS and iliac crest heights are expected to reflect torsional effects, PSIS asymmetry (discussed in the next paragraph) will be a more sensitive measure.

It is tempting to expect that in the case of anatomic LLI, the unleveling of the iliac crests would be identical to the unleveling of the PSISs: i.e, that lines drawn though the highest points of the iliac crests and through the PSISs would be parallel on an x-ray. In fact, there is no guarantee this would occur, because anatomic LLI may result in pelvic torsion. Although this is explained in detail in the next chapter, suffice it to say for the current discussion that the innominate bone often rotates anteriorly on the side of an anatomic short leg, so that the lines mentioned above would not be parallel.

Note simultaneous palpation of iliac crests and PSISs.

Look and feel of the PSISs

PSIS palpation is more difficult than one would think. We believe the best method involves grasping both innominates, with the fingers on the crests while the thumbs reach over and feel for the PSISs. The examiner really does require the tactile sense of the entire hand to feel confidence in identifying the PSIS. In a research setting, we draw horizontal lines across the thumb nail, and use a rule or tape to measure the heights of these horizontal lines from the floor. A

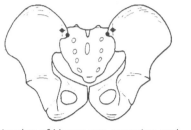

Dimples of Venus are superior and lateral to PSISs. Note depth also.

How "dimple lag" was discovered.

clinician, in a real clinical setting, cannot easily do that, and will thus have to rely on the visual appearance of the thumbs. If left-right vertical asymmetry is hard to determine, it probably isn't large enough to be worth determining.

The PSIS, like the iliac crest, is lower on the posteriorly rotated innominate bone, "all other things being equal" – in other words, if there is no confounding anatomic LLI. It feels more prominent for two reasons: first, the relative anteriority of the sacrum leaves the PSIS less surrounded with soft tissue; second, the PSIS can be felt to be more posterior because the AP measurement of the cleaved innominate bone is increased. As already noted, PSIS palpation is more sensitive than innominate crest palpation for pelvic torsion. If there is anatomic LLI, sitting PSIS palpation is of paramount significance in identifying torsional states, as we discuss below in the section of sitting examination findings. Indeed, we can not interpret standing PSIS heights minus the information from the sitting examination.

Some clinicians claim they can palpate the distance between the PSIS and the second sacral tubercle, and that the measurement is decreased on the side of posterior pelvic cleavage, owing to the fact that the innominate bone swings medially as well when it cleaves. My own calculations indicate that this is unlikely, in that the amount by which the innominate swings medially is very small in relation to the amount by which it travels posteroinferiorly.

Sacroiliac visualization

The sacroiliac "dimple" that lies just superolateral to the PSIS that is will appear more obvious (deeper). Not all patients have dimples that can be easily visualized. Sometimes subtle differences in shading make a difference in terms of how well the dimples can be seen. Apart from appearing deeper, the dimple ought to be inferior consistent with the PSIS on that same side of the body.

On another note, there has been research on the curious phenomenon of "dimple lag": if one foot of a standing patient is elevated by a known amount by inserting something under it, the ipsilateral dimple raises up by a smaller amount.[3] The authors inferred from this finding that there had to be pelvic torsion, which reduced the amount the innominate would rise when the ipsilateral foot is elevated. Another article, using an optoelectric measuring device instead of dimple visualization, came to the same conclusions.

Lumbosacral hyperextension and true hyperlordosis

The lumbosacral joint and/or L4-5 may be hyperextended, with the rest of the lumbar spine being relatively *hypolordotic*; or the entire lumbopelvis may be involved in a hyperlordotic curve. I refer to these alternative states as hyperextension and hyperlordosis, respectively. These particular faults, not surprisingly, indicate what may as well be called "deimbrication" moves. The doctor applies a thrust in the vicinity of the sacral apex and/or the ischial tuberosities, so as to flex the lumbosacral joint at least, and to a lesser extent some of the superior motor units. This is not advised for patients thought to be at risk of having or sustaining a disc herniation, who need flexion plus rotation about as much as they need a hole in the head. Apart from the side-posture thrusting procedures, there are other ways of flattening the hyperlordotic lumbopelvis, such as supine and prone drop-table moves as described by Thompson and others; moreover, there are procedures using padded wedges as well (in a separate chapter, below).

Lumbar hypolordosis and flattening of the sacral base angle

The hypolordotic patient presents a special problem, in that long term increased weight bearing on the anterior spinal joints (the IVDs) seems to be associated with discopathy. This is certainly the case with acute IVD syndrome, or herniated disc. We would not want to introduce forces that would further flex the patient and increase posterior discal pressure. (The case of flexion-distraction technique, or "distraction technique" as it now appears to be called, is worthy of discussion at this point, but we resist the temptation in order to avoid being distracted.) Adjustive procedures that extend the lumbosacral area make more sense, including a sacral base contact on the long leg side, a PI ilium short lever move,

Drerup B, Hierholzer E. Movement of the human pelvis and displacement of related anatomical landmarks on the body surface. J Biomech 1987;20(10):971-7.

and low segmental lumbar moves. Here we are in the world of classic "thou shalt not rotate" Gonstead. In a sense, as we move from the hyperextended to the hyperflexed low back patient, we also move from Pettibonesque deimbrication maneuvers to those of Gonstead, on the basis of both their intrinsic mechanical propriety and issues of patient safety. All clinicians should learn to cohabit both of these adjustive universes.

Linear translations

An anterolisthesis is, of course, an anterior slippage of L5 (very often the entirety of the lumbar spine) on the sacral base. We note the difference between a spondylolytic spondylolisthesis and a nonspondylolisthetic (degenerative) spondylolisthesis. The lines of correction for translatory distortions are mostly obvious, flowing directly from the description of the subluxation: thrust P to A on L5 for a retro of L5, or A to P on S1 for an anterolisthesis of L5. But even here there is wiggle room. Pettibon and some of his followers have favored a side-posture manipulative approach in which a thrust is applied near the sacral apex on a patient who is placed in extreme lumbothoracic kyphosis. The idea is that this would tighten up the posterior longitudinal ligament, and thus tend to straighten up George's line, in effect, realigning the lower lumbar and sacral segments. Interestingly enough, this all-purpose sacral apex move would benefit anterolisthesis or retrolistheses of either L4 or L5.

We have very little to say about lateralistheses, except to say they occur, often in individuals whose case provides an explanation for such an obvious sign of instability: old age, poor nutrition, trauma, congenital hypermobility, inflammatory arthritis, etc. In many cases, thrusting techniques would not be indicated, and less forceful techniques such as mobilization and soft tissue treatment would be more likely to get a good and safe outcome.

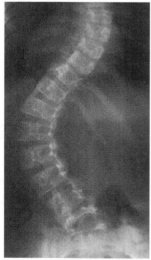

Scoliosis

By "scoliosis" we do not confine our discussion to severe cases of idiopathic juvenile scoliosis, and understand the term to include the less dramatic cases of spinal curvature that chiropractors routinely see. We do not, on the other hand, think it defensible to apply the term to a lateral flexion malposition of one vertebra in relation to the subjacent one, as we see it done sometimes.

We accept as a truism, although it has not been clinically verified to our knowledge, that adjustive strategies that have the effect of opening the concave side of the scoliotic spine make sense, as compared with, let's say, a strategy of increasing the degree of concavity. Although some clinicians, in thrusting from the convex side of the curvature, have the goal of reducing or eliminating the curvature, and although we would certainly not turn down any such improvement in a scoliotic patient, it need not be our primary goal. Rather, we simply claim that the outcome of care is likely to be better if thrusts are delivered that would distract the tissues on the concave side, and approximate those on the convex side, even if the bones wind up exactly where they started prior to the thrust. This is, of course, a testable hypothesis that has not been to our knowledge tested. We might add that in cases of scoliosis. It is tempting to speculate as to the putative benefits of this strategy, which amounts to adjusting "as if" you could reduce scoliosis, even when you suspect you can't; but we will resist that temptation for the moment.

Although we are discussing lateral curvature, we cannot leave the discussion without making the analogous comment for the sagittal plane. Patients often exhibit increased and/or decreased kyphoses and lordoses. Indeed, often the same patient will show both, as when a hyperextended cervical spine is associated with a hyperkyphotic upper thoracic spine. We apply the "as if" strategy here as well: try to flatten the hyperkyphoses, and flex the hyperextensions. The reasoning is the same. Even without achieving discernible alterations in the sagittal posture, we believe the patient is made better off by having, even for just a moment in time, the contractured soft tissues elongated, their adhesions torn, pain-spasm-pain cycles interrupted, pathological neurological reflex loops blocked, and so on. Proof? You want proof? So do I! But in the meantime, we will have to go with what seems more plausible, compared with other hypotheses.

Lateral bending of L4 on L5

It is very common to have L5 "follow suit" with the pelvis, and yet have L4 strike an unexpected position with respect to L5. After all, L5 is closely tethered to the ilium by the iliolumbar ligament, and L4-5 has more freedom to get into trouble. Indeed, as advance imaging becomes more and more affordable, we are beginning to discern a huge number of disc problems at L4-5,

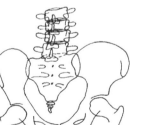

Normal subject x-rayed in right rotation, creating false impression of Lovett-reverse (from Hildebrandt)

Tortipelvis, with anomalous open wedge on concave side of spine (from Barge).

perhaps even more than at L5-S1. In going over a few examples of anomalous L4-5 configurations, we must realize we have departed from the land of the Basic Distortion, and are swimming in uncharted, or rather poorly charted, waters. It's the world of segmentalism, where (almost) anything can happen, that world that seems so familiar to chiropractors and yet has been so challenging from a clinical point of view: poor reproducibility of exam findings, poor correspondence of exam findings to symptoms, etc. Personally, I prefer predictive models to "whatever is, is" (i.e., segmental) clinical situations. Segmental subluxations, their apparent arbitrariness notwithstanding, should be addressed as such.

A number of things can go wrong at L4-5, many of which take the form of a divergent disc angle on an otherwise convex side of the spine. Dr. Barge terms cases such as these tortipelvis. The pelvis and L5 may be relatively level, while L4-5 begins a rotatory scoliosis to one side or the other. Or the pelvis and L5 may be inferior on one side, while L4-5 absurdly decides to initiate a lateral curvature, convex on the opposite side! This is the so-called Lovett-reverse configuration, but caution is urged in overinterpreting radiographs that seem to demonstrate this "subluxation." As Hildebrandt shows in his excellent text *Chiropractic Spinography*[4], a normal subject who is radiographed while even slightly turned on the Y axis, given full spine radiography, would appear to have this Lovett-reverse configuration, even though this conclusion would be entirely bogus. Finally, we sometimes see that the lumbar spine is *excessively* convex on the same side as a low sacrum, beginning at L4, with a so-called "open wedge" at L4-5 on the otherwise concave side of the spine.

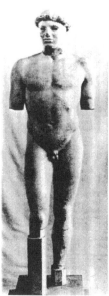

Ignore anatomic LLI in this sculpture.

Posterior spine and lateral flank appearance

There may be an obvious lateral curvature of the lumbar spine, as determined by spinous process palpation and visualization. It helps to put water-soluble marks on the spinous processes. This can be done in the prone position more easily, but one expects diminution of the lateral curvature when the patient is no longer upright; in that case, it is very helpful to sight the skin marks by getting low and looking up the long axis of the table from the foot of the table. The lumbar musculature can be seen and palpated to be more posterior on the side of posterior pelvic cleavage. This is owing to the fact that the spinous processes in general turn toward the concave side of spinal lateral curvatures, which is to say the vertebral bodies turn toward the

Hildebrandt RW. Chiropractic Spinography. 2nd ed. Baltimore: Williams & Wilkins; 1985.

convex side. This carries the transverse processes and the overlaying soft tissue posteriorly, a result that can be seen and felt.

The flank can be visualized to be more convex on the side of posterior pelvic cleavage by virtue of the fact that the lumbothoracic spine forms a convexity on this same side. The contralateral flank by comparison appears either straight or possibly concave. The rather inglorious expression "love handles" adequately describes the flank on the side of anterior pelvic cleavage. There may be an increased distance between one of the hanging arms and the flank, confirming spinal concavity on that side. Although it may be the case that lateral curvature of the lumbar spine, with an associated opposite curvature of the thoracic spine, may be a normal variant, at least to a certain extent, we would still want to take such curvatures into account when considering possible lines of drive once the decision to intervene has been made on clinical grounds. In other words, the clinician may not feel it appropriate to attempt straightening the spine of an asymptomatic subject, but once a patient has developed signs of dysfunction, the presence of lateral curvature would certainly bear on the choice of adjustive strategies. Most commonly, forces are applied from lateral to medial on the side of spinal convexity, so as to "close the open wedge."

Anatomic leg length inequality

We have already discussed in detail the import of anatomic LLI. In order to compensate for a structural short leg and resultant inferiority of the sacral base, the pelvis may rotate posteriorly on the long leg side, and anterior on the short leg side. The iliac crest may even wind up higher in the standing position on the posteriorly rotated side, and as we have seen, the functional short leg side in the prone exam may be challenging to interpret.

James Dean standing comfort test

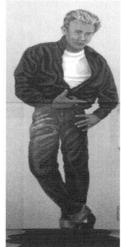

The act of standing, far from being a simple thing, is actually quite complicated and involves alternating between left and right-sided slouches. See the discussion in the chapter *On Standing*. If one were to recall the image of the rebel without a cause, especially the famous movie still in which the stooped Dean contemptuously smokes a cigarette clad in cuffed denim (Dean is clad and cuffed, not the cigarette) and turned up collar, it evokes quite accurately the body language of pelvic torsion. This is how a person "sits on himself" in the standing position (as TEO used to put it); that is, bears more weight on the one leg at the expense of the other, which is carried with the knee bent. The patient is asked to slouch "like James Dean," first with one knee bent and then with the other (the legs need not be actually crossed, as in the figure of Dean), which in reality has the patient assuming alternately a left and then a right PI configuration.

One side of slouch will feel more comfortable or at least natural for the patient. Although an unusual patient may complain of outright pain in the rib cage, foot, knee, hip, or back, more often than not, there is a vague sense of something not feeling quite right. If the patient prefers bearing weight on the right leg (is a "right Dean") this translates to a left PI syndrome, and vice versa. This clinical regimen is actually a particular example of an orthopedic procedure which is called an "apprehension test," for example the test for patellar stability which entails watching the patient's face for signs of apprehension while the examiner puts lateral pressure on the patella. We have already asked the reader to try clasping the hands opposite to the usual manner, and reasoned that if there is a preferred pattern of hand clasping, departure from which feels distinctly abnormal, there should be nothing puzzling about the fact that there is a preferred standing slouch pattern.

Torso rotation

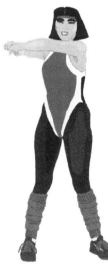

The standing patient is asked to clasp his hands at the in front of the chest and then rotate the torso to the end point of motion, first to the left and then to the right. One direction will subjectively feel to the patient more comfortable or exhibit less strain at the end point than the other. This will be the same side as that to which the patient normally and spontaneously spins his torso in order to self-treat a stiff and/or painful back, usually producing an audible release. It turns out that the patient turns more easily toward the side of the posterior innominate cleavage. I believe, but am not certain, that this result would also obtain for many subjects who carry their pelvis inferiorly due to anatomic LLI; but the matter is confounded by the possibility of torsional compensation for the structural asymmetry.

Turning toward the posteriorly rotated side of the pelvis unwinds the helical component of the torsion syndrome: each lumbopelvic segment is anterior with respect to the segment below on the side of the PI; therefore, twisting the torso from the shoulders down rotates each segment posteriorly with respect to the segment below, undoing the distortion. A moment's reflection will in addition establish another interesting corollary: a patient turning toward his posteriorly cleaved innominate bone is in reality accomplishing a self-adjustment akin to a garden variety PI ilium adjustment - the shoulder is thrust posteriorly, and the same side hip is kept relatively anterior by virtue of the fixed position of the feet on the floor.

Let us note that many chiropractors, historically and to this day, routinely perform a move called by some the "million dollar roll," a side-posture manipulative maneuver that produces marked counter-rotation of the pelvic and shoulder girdles. Although it has become fashionable to denounce such maneuvers as being from the chiropractic "stone age," one will hear no such denunciation from this author. It is important to remember, in conceptualizing the patient's overall lumbopelvic distortion, that the helical winding of the lumbar spine is every bit as much a component as any other factor that can be identifed, just as important as, let us say, the inferiority of the sacral base or posterior rotation of the innominate bone. I would suggest only that chiropractors, in performing their rolls, cut it back to perhaps a "fifty dollar roll"; that they perform it on only one side, that of posterior innominate rotation, so they don't worsen the helix; and that they employ a contact hand to isolate out the most restricted segment and constitute it as a fixed point in-between the contrary rotations of the shoulder and pelvic girdles.

There is another clinical point worth making here. If the patient complains of excessive back or rib cage pain while being pre-positioned for a side posture manipulative procedure, due consideration should be given to a couple of possibilities. If the doctor intends the PI side to be up, then the doctor's listing may simply be wrong. If the doctor intends the AS side to be up, it is to be expected, since the pre-stress worsens the helix, that the patient would experience some degree of discomfort. The doctor can minimize this by reducing the amount of rotation, and indeed, should do this. One thing for sure: whether the listing is right or wrong, patient apprehension is a real deal-killer when it comes to manipulative procedures.

Thoracic spine appearance and palpation

The thoracolumbar spine forms an s-shaped scoliosis, with the lumbar portion convex on the side of the posterior innominate cleavage, and the thoracic spine convex on the opposite side. In cases where the lumbar spine is hard to visualize or palpate, it may be easier to *infer* its structure from the more easily discerned structure of the thoracic spine. Obviously, it is always better to palpate the lumbar spine as compared with inferring anything about its structure, but we must remember to always be realistic: if the palpatory procedure is of questionable reproducibility, and the evidence is not overwhelming anyway, then one would have more confidence in predicting the lumbar spine from a very clear read on the thoracic spine.

Given that the thoracic spine may exhibit more superiorly a second curvature opposite in its direction from its first curvature, it is important that the examiner ascertain that she or he has truly detected the first thoracic compensation to the lumbar convexity. These curvatures can be palpated, and can also be directly visualized in which case the task is made easier if the spinous processes are marked with a wax pencil. As discussed above, the identification of thoracic lateral curvature is likely to affect the line of drive, once the decision to intervene has been made on clinical grounds.

Taut sacrospinalis and quadratus lumborum muscles

On the side of posterior innominate cleavage, the sacrospinalis group of the erector spinae muscles will enter into hypertonic contraction in a vain attempt to elevate the sacrum. Likewise, the quadratus lumborum muscle, taking origin from the 12th rib and the transverse processes of L1-4 and inserting on the iliac crest, will attempt to elevate the iliac crest. These hypertonic muscle states may be palpated by comparing the tissue compliance on either side of the spine at about the level of L4, lateral to the spine. It is recommended that the examiner use the same finger on a given hand rather than a different finger from each hand, in order to rule out variation in his or her own bilateral proprioceptive sense in assessment of the relative tissue compliance.

Lower extremity posture and function

The lower extremity findings vary according to whether we allow the subject to stand "as usual" or have the subject take on that more rigid stance they assume whenever in front of a doctor with a clipboard. Some of the findings, such as pronation and foot flare, would be about the same, whereas others would likely disappear, such as hip and knee flexion. The most significant change is in weight distribution between the left and right legs.

There may be a tendency to show increased hip and/or knee flexion on the side of posterior innominate rotation, according to Dr. Logan, with whom we agree. These changes could also be obtained as the consequence of an ipsilateral structural long leg, for reasons that are intuitively obvious. Therefore, we should not try to interpret any such observations, in a relaxed subject, minus all the other examination findings (including compressive leg checking and sitting PSIS determination). That stated, there are

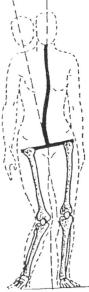

Note pronation, valgus knee, inferior pelvis, spinal curvature.

some findings that are worthy of being noted. The figure shows several of the relationships in question. Note the increased valgus angle of the knee, the pronated foot, the medial tibial rotation in relation to the foot, medial rotation of the femur in relation to the tibia, and the external rotation of the entire leg (at the hip, of course). These individual items are discussed below.

Foot carriage

In the standing position the foot is externally rotated, or exhibits toe-out. It is better to observe the patient unaware, rather than instructing "stand as you always stand," which is impossible under such artificial circumstances. The foot is externally rotated as an indirect consequence of the sacral apex being deviated away from the side of the lowered sacral base, whether the result of pelvic torsion or anatomical LLI. The piriformis muscle, an important lateral rotator of the leg, originates from three lips on the anterior side of the sacral border, the margin of the greater sciatic foramen, and the sacrotuberous ligament. It passes through the sciatic foramen to insert on the superior border of the greater trochanter. On the side of the lowered pelvis, the piriformis muscle will become hypertonic in a vain attempt to pull over the sacral apex which has deviated contralaterally. Although the sacral apex deviation cannot be undone, because the subject (after all) presents with this asymmetric posture, the piriformis does wind up laterally rotating the entire lower extremity.

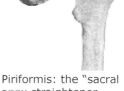

Piriformis: the "sacral apex straightener outer"muscle.

The foot will also tend to be pronated, as evidenced by eversion of the calcaneus and an inward bowing of the achilles tendon. The examiner slides a finger under the longitudinal arch of each foot, and finds that the finger encounters more resistance on the side of the innominate posteriority. The subject will also confirm increased tenderness of the calcaneonavicular ("spring") ligament on this same side. There are postural reasons to expect the other foot to be pronated as well, possibly to a similar extent. This means that the finding of a pronated foot does not rule in a PI distortion on the same side, but the absence of a pronated foot would certainly argue against there being PI pelvic torsion. This amounts to saying that the pronation is sensitive for, but not especially specific for, posterior pelvic torsion. Individuals with genu varum may stand with a normal foot posture, or even with supination; however, their underlying pronation would manifest during walking or running (see Management of Common Musculoskeletal Disorders, Hertling and Kessler, 2nd ed. p.400.).

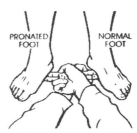

Taken from *Foot Levelers* literature.

Knee carriage

The knee on the side of posterior cleavage is slightly bent, in order to accommodate to the physiological "lengthening" of the leg that is brought about by the acetabulum being carried inferiorly. Lateral tibial torsion, to be expected with increased foot flare, is associated with an increased valgus angle in the knee. Furthermore, the femur is medially rotated with respect to the tibia, increasing the Q-angle of the knee (the valgus angle is accentuated). Pronation of the ipsilateral foot also adds to the increased valgus angle of the knee. It is not likely that this could be easily palpated or measured, barring an x-ray.

The symptoms of pain and/or tenderness at the medial aspect of the knee are also easily demonstrated in the supine position. There will be tenderness or frank pain at the pes anserine bursa, the medial collateral ligament, and/or the medial meniscus due to the increased valgus angle on the side of the lowered pelvis. There is abnormal stretch placed on those muscles which span the distance between the innominate bone and the knee: sartorius, rectus femoris, and gracilis. Sartorius is especially stretched, by the valgus angle increase in addition to the posterior innominate rotation, if there is pelvic torsion at the root of the distortion. The muscles engage in a futile attempt to reduce the knee flexion and/or posterior carriage of the innominate bone, eventually becoming tender at their insertion at the pes anserine bursa.

Weight-bearing

Although it would not be a very expensive investment, most doctors do not keep a pair of scales in the office that could be used to measure bilateral weight distribution. Dr. Hugh Logan claimed a patient bore more weight on the side of posterior innominate rotation, even though I have claimed above that the patient bears more weight on the side of anterior innominate rotation, when there is pelvic torsion. The paradox is easily resolved: the rigid stance of the patient knowing he or she is being observed shows more weight on the PI side, as Dr. Logan indicated, whereas the relaxed standing pose shows more weight on the anterior rotation side.

The situation of anatomic LLI is more complicated, there being some data to the effect that whether more weight is borne on the short or long leg side depends on the amount of the inequality.

Prone leg checking

Leg checking is so distinctive that it warrants its own chapter. Please see below.

The PSIS has already been observed and palpated in the standing position. In the prone position the PSIS once again feels more prominent, because the relative anteriority of the sacrum leaves it less surrounded with soft tissue and because the AP measurement of the cleaved innominate bone is increased. Again, the distance between the PSIS and the second sacral tubercle is *very slightly* decreased on the side of posterior pelvic cleavage, so slightly that one wonders if most differences are truly palpable. It is typical that the inferior PSIS in the standing position reverses to become the superior PSIS prone. This results from the hypertonic musculature that is futile at elevating the low hip in the standing position, but effective in the prone or supine position, barring excessive friction at the patient-table interface.

There is, however, no guarantee of standing-prone reversal of the PSIS positions. There are two competing influences on the PSIS position: posterior pelvic torsion renders it more *caudal*, while the pull of the hypertonic suprapelvic muscles (quadratus lumborum, sacrospinalis) laterally flexes the pelvis, pulling the PSIS *cephalad* on the side of the standing low hip. The net result is indeterminate, but usually the muscle pull effect overcomes the torsional effect, so that the prone PSIS is cephalad.

Carriage of the sacrum

The lateral borders of the sacrum and the sacral apex can be directly and easily palpated, enabling the examiner to ascertain the position of the sacrum with respect to the crease between the buttocks. The sacral apex will be noted to be deviated laterally away from the side of the posterior innominate cleavage. More often than not the lateral border of the sacrum can be felt to have rotated anteriorly on the side of posterior cleavage.

When there is pelvic torsion, the posterior rotation of the innominate bone leaves the sacral base in a relatively anterior position at the sacroiliac joint. This can be palpated as follows: the examiner uses the thumbs to locate the left and right PSISs, and then simply roll off of them, medially, into the sacroiliac joint. Here we have to be careful, because the palpatory procedure detects both the comparative *depth* of the right and left SI joints, in addition to the comparative *position* of the left and right sides of the sacral base.

The thumb sinks more easily into the deeper SI joint, on the side of sacral base anteriority; that is, the SI joint is "deeper." On the other hand, since the sacral base was carried posteriorly with the innominate bone on the side of posterior innominate rotation, it will be more posterior with respect to the other side of the sacrum. Therefore, we are left with the following paradox: the sacral base is palpated anterior to the same-side innominate bone, but posterior with respect to the opposite side of the sacrum. This probably accounts for the discrepancy between chiropractors who agree the sacrum is inferior, but disagree whether it is at the same time posterior (e.g, Gonstead clinicians) or anterior (e.g., Logan and Thompson technique clinicians).

Muscle function and pelvic torsion

The gluteus maximus and the hamstring muscles are chronically stretched on the side of anterior hemipelvic rotation; the gluteus maximus by the anterosuperior drift of the innominate bone away from the posterior aspect of the femur, and the hamstrings by the elevation of the ischial tuberosity away from the knee. These muscles are weak because they are in a state of consequent stretch weakness (this terminology is borrowed from Kendall and McCreary[5]), and are demonstrably weak on manual muscle testing. The gluteus maximus is tested by having the patient extend the thigh against examiner resistance, the

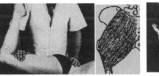

Dr. Walther, testing gluteus maximus.

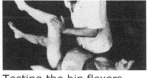

Testing the hip flexors, attempting to isolate rectus femoris.

hamstrings by having her flex the bent knee against resistance. The hamstrings will not generally manifest weakness unless the test is initiated from an angle of about 25 degrees.

The rectus femoris and sartorius, insofar as each originates on the innominate bone and inserts near the knee joint, are both stretched by the posterior rotation of the innominate bone. They will be found to exhibit stretch weakness upon manual muscle testing. The rectus femoris muscle is tested by having the supine patient perform a resisted thigh flexion, starting with the hip and knee at 90 degrees. The sartorius is less easily tested, and would not normally need to be tested in the event that the rectus femoris demonstrated a clear pattern. Probably the psoas muscle would also be found weak on the side of posterior torsion, but I have not been checking this muscle systematically over the years, so I can not say for sure that it is weak.

I used to think that this muscle weakness resulted from a histologically-verifiable degeneration of the lengthened muscle, and indeed it is not hard to find citations

Kendall HO, Kendall FP, Wadsworth GE. Muscle testing and function. 2nd ed. Baltimore, MD: Williams & Wilkins; 1971.

to that effect. However, the clinical finding that the strength of these muscles may be at least temporarily restored immediately upon an intervention, be it soft tissue or manipulative, casts some doubt on our impression that the underlying phenomenon is myofascial, or histological in nature. Careful observation of the subject during the procedure of manual muscle testing suggests that there is more difficulty *marshaling* the body's resources in resisting the examiner's stretching force; the subject's leg can be seen to wobble in anticipation of the test, which renders resistance more difficult. It's as though there is some level of unconscious fear of weakness, that is manifested as something of a self-fulfilling prophecy. Finally, would it be too much of a stretch to say that this muscle weakness is a matter of "nerve interference" – not an actin/myosin problem, but one of neuromusculoskeletal control?

Pelvic torsion challenge sign

The author employs a version of the "vertebral challenge," as described in the chapter entitled "The Clinical Evidence," to determine not only the pattern of pelvic torsion, but also which sacroiliac joint is the "involved side," i.e., the "major." The only other part of the spine I routinely evaluate that way is the atlanto-occipital joint, not because I believe that the only other joint amenable to such evaluation, but because I reserve the right to be a creature of habit.

The presence of pelvic torsion gives rise to a reflex phenomenon that can be detected using a procedure that is described by Applied Kinesiologists [6], called the vertebral challenge. It is first necessary to select a muscle that can be shown to be strong by manual muscle testing, the hamstrings with the knee flexed at 90 degrees serving quite well in the prone position. The examiner applies a *very mild* thrust – a low velocity, low amplitude thrust – to one PSIS and the contralateral ischium (toward a presumed line of correction), and then immediately retests the "previously strong indicator muscle" (PSIM). If the muscle weakens, it is inferred that there is posterior pelvic cleavage on the side of the PSIS that was contacted, and the contralateral side is anteriorly cleaved. If on the other hand the PSIM remains strong, then the examiner presents an opposite pattern of challenge to the body, while the PSIM is rechecked to see if the other innominate bone instead is relatively posteriorly cleaved.

Although it is certainly counterintuitive, muscle weakness is interpreted as follows: if a proposed line of drive would indeed correct a problem, the body's way of saying "Yes, please adust me just that way" is that a test muscle weakens.

Walther DS. Applied Kinesiology, Volume I. Pueblo, Colorado: Systems DC; 1981.

Walther explains, citing osteopath Sutherland for the point, that the test thrust stretches and further provokes shortened muscles; which causes reflex stimulation of these muscles owing to stretch reflexes; which pulls the bone into a state of greater misalignment "on the rebound"; which in some way results in a momentary generalized muscle weakness. There are clearly elements of genius in this, but also possible *hooey*, in that it is not obvious why a state of increased lesion, if indeed that happens, would cause a generalized weakness. On the other hand, I would not be spending any time on this if I did not think the effect real, whatever the ultimate explanation turns out to be.

It may be illustrative to compare and contrast the challenge with a more vigorous thrust. By comparison, this would be a high velocity, low amplitude thrust. As explained by Sandoz[7] and others, our working model is that a manipulative thrust, when aimed in the direction that would reduce a misalignment or at least stretch spasmed muscles, causes muscle inhibition by means of activating the Golgi Tendon Organ. This results in a better state of joint alignment and/or function. It may be that the thrust at first activates the spindle fibers (stretch reflex), increasing the load on the GTO, increasing the likelihood that it will exert its inhibitory effect on the musculature.

What about a low velocity, low amplitude "thrust" perpetrated for a long time, much longer than that seen in the challenge procedure? That would amount to traction, of which multiple types abound in chiropractic: blocking with padded wedges, using pillows under the patient, setting table tops in inclined positions, etc. It is commonly said that stretching (traction) relaxes muscles, stretches out contracted ligamentous tissue, quiets down neurological reflex loops, and so on.

Provocative lumbopelvic testing with padded wedges

The diagnostic and therapeutic use of padded wedges is so important that it receives its own chapter later in the text, but a shor comment here might be worth the trouble

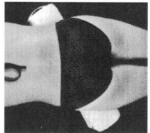

Padded wedges, as popularized by SOT practitioners, are positioned under the patient in a manner thought to reverse the apparent pelvic torsion. A high block is inserted under the superior aspect of the iliac crest on the presumed AS side, and a low block under the acetabular region on the presumed PI side. If there is pain or tenderness in either of

Prone blocking with padded wedges.

Sandoz R. Some physical mechanisms and effects of spinal adjustments. Annals of the Swiss Chiropractic Association 1976;6:91-141.

the SI joints or the lumbar spine, it is aggravated by incorrect blocking, and ameliorated by correct blocking. (Of course, if the wedges are simply left in place for a measured period of time, this "diagnostic procedure" becomes a treatment procedure.) The wedges can also be used to track down double PI (hypolordotic) patients, and double AS (hyperlordotic) patients as well.

There are 8 ways to perform provocative pelvic blocking: high left, low right; low left, high right; double high; double low; high left single block; high right single block; low left single block; and low right single block. These pain provocative/ameliorative procedures amount to a form of orthopedic testing, since the purpose of virtually any such test is to put the joint under investigation in a stressed or de-stressed position, noting whatever symptomatic changes there are and drawing the obvious conclusion as to the mechanical derangement which is thereby evidenced. The results of provocative blocking may accrue to the aggravation/amelioration of *fixation patterns* in addition to or instead of the positional theory evinced in this section of the text, and this is discussed in the chapter on blocking (below). Moreover, a case is made that from a treatment point of view, it may not be that important to decide if the blocking results dictate any particular mechanical "listing"; rather, the blocking results permit the practitioner to directly decide upon the adjustive strategy, regarding the lumbopelvis as something of a black box.

Sacral leg check

The patient is asked to extend the thigh with the knee held straight, while the examiner applies firm pressure to the sacral base. (Dr. 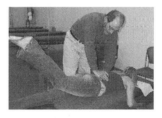 Thompson, who originally described this sign, recommends that the examiner stabilize the sacral base with his fingers pointed inferiorly, but I find the stabilization to be more effective and the test to be more reliable if the fingers are directed up the spine.) The leg does not extend as far or perhaps extends more slowly and painfully on the side of posterior innominate cleave. This results from the fact that the subject has a tendency to hold his thigh somewhat flexed on the side of the posterior innominate bone, which results in chronic contracture of the anterior iliofemoral tissues: both the ligaments, including the hip capsule, and the thigh flexor muscles (sartorius, rectus femoris, and psoas). This soft tissue shortening restricts thigh extension. Furthermore, leg extension tends to rotate the innominate bone posteriorly, which will be resisted by whatever entities (articular, muscular) that have been responsible for the posterior torsion in the first place.

This test can seem frustrating, since it is uncommon to attain the same test result in a second doing. Rather than reducing the credibility of the test, this variability argues *in favor of* its validity. This is a *destructive test*, meaning it destroys the evidence it is designed to detect. Leg raising stretches the soft tissue contractures, so it is likely that a repetition of the procedure will manifest less reduction in the range of motion.

A moment's reflection should establish the fact that the sacral leg check, as described by Thompson, is equivalent to the supine procedure described in the field of medical orthopedics as the Thomas test, which detects psoas tightening. Actually, there is no such thing as "medical" or "chiropractic" orthopedics, just orthopedic tests that are indigenous to one field or another, but which enter the common domain in often overlapping manners.

Pain

The pain may result from a lumbar segmental joint, a sacroiliac joint, the iliolumbar ligament, or any of the muscle bellies, and so on. In addition to everything else, pelvic torsion *may* indeed hurt. Levangie, having measured several sitting and standing parameters she thought indicative of pelvic torsion, failed to find much evidence that any of them predicted lumbopelvic pain.[8] That is somewhat troubling, but represents only a modest setback for those of us who suppose clinical signs of pelvic torsion bear implications for adjustive vectors. After all, at least for those of us who largely deal with symptomatic patients, the question isn't so much whether torsion tends to cause pain, but whether the finding of torsion suggests reasonable lines of drive in treating a patient who is in pain thought to be related to torsion. By analogy, hypertension need not hurt, but when a patient presents with chronic headache attributable to hypertension, that condition had best be treated.

Sometimes there is frank pain and other times there is merely tenderness to palpation. Certainly the pain sometimes indicates a hypermobile compensation for a primary (usually contralateral) hypomobile subluxation. However, the point is often overdone. It is our clinical impression, and we have seen a little evidence to this effect, that pain and tenderness usually identify *restricted* joints. Of course, torn and stretched ligaments that result in hypermobility produce pain as well. We just have to be on our guard against adopting rules like "pain doesn't matter, we are interested only in 'objective indicators' of subluxation"; and the equally silly "pain means a joint is hypermobile, leave it alone."

Levangie PK. The association between static pelvic asymmetry and low back pain. Spine 1999;24(12):1234-42.

Pain and/or tenderness represent only one of a number of local findings that may be obtained in the prone position. Each of the intervertebral posterior joints should be individually checked for springiness, as some have called it, amounting to the assessment of joint end-feel: is it hard, or is there access to the paraphysiological joint space? If the doctor has lit upon a posterior joint restriction, the patient can usually confirm that the joint is tender to the touch. Indeed, it might be the patient's response to the provocative pressure, muscle splinting or something even more subtle, that the doctor identifies as "fixation." In addition to palpating the quality of joint movements, the doctor may also identify soft tissue textural changes. The flesh often feels firm and somewhat thickened above posterior joints that are dysfunctional, as can be confirmed with a skin rolling maneuver in which the doctor ascends the spine while gathering the flesh bilaterally between the thumb and index finger. Obviously, this palpatory procedure is more easily demonstrated than described in a text!

Appendix: Assessing sacral base rotation

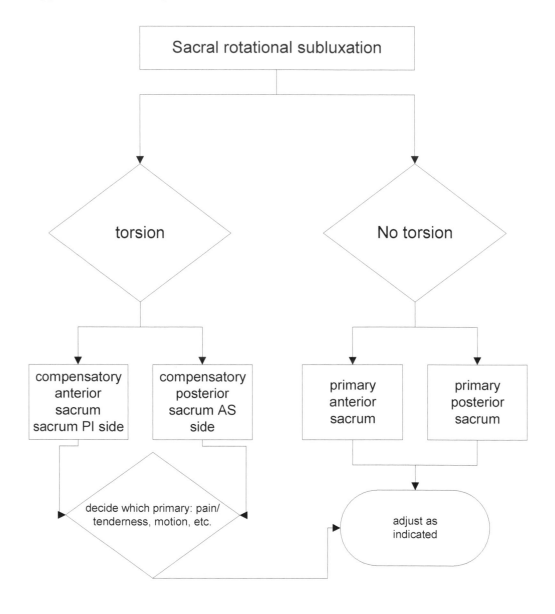

8. Chiropractic leg checking

Having gone through the pathological anatomy of the lumbopelvis, we next turn to the examination findings that would be expected of patients, those with and without the pelvic torsion syndrome that we have so heavily emphasized. We are going to go over standing, sitting, supine, and prone findings. The leg check, one of a series of examination procedures performed usually in the prone position, should be considered in due course when we get to the section on prone findings. However, given the central (almost sacred!) importance of leg checking, the author has decided to cut right to the quick and deal with the matter – what the leg check *does* and *does not* identify – in its own standalone chapter. It is really worth a standalone *book*, but that is a project that will have to wait for some future time.

Chiropractors, physical therapists, and osteopaths all seem fairly obsessed with the short leg syndrome, partly because asymmetry of the lower extremities is thought to have painful consequences for the patient, and partly because it is thought to have diagnostic significance. In chiropractic, leg checking is used in a number of circumstances:

• to illuminate the status of the atlanto-occipital joint

• to provide a window into pelvic torsion

• to serve as an outcome measure following provocative procedures, like cervical rotation (Derifield cervical check), and like isolation testing (Activator technique);

• as an outcome measure to track the patient's short and long term response to chiropractic adjustive care.

One is hard pressed to know exactly what is going through a person's mind when doing his or her first leg check, but one supposes the thought, however transiently, must arise that a leg that looks shorter than the other one, well, may be shorter! In other words, sometimes things may seem as simple as they are. Under what circumstances would it make sense to assume that legs that seem uneven are actually the same length, but in different distal positions due to a state of subluxation in the pelvis, upper cervical area, or any other region of the body? Remember, several investigators have found that as many as half of normal subjects, and a larger proportion of symptomatic subjects, have anatomic leg length inequality of a quarter inch or more.[1]

Chiropractic leg checking, perhaps first popularized by Dr. Mabel Derifield, has served as one of the primary chiropractic diagnostic inputs and output measures for many decades. The respect afforded leg checking by those who have grown accustomed to its use is exceeded only by the scorn of the skeptics, who find it bizarre that any thinking person, let alone a doctor, would find it useful to carefully inspect the feet, when the patient, after all, complains of neck or back pain. Strong opinions notwithstanding, very little quantitative or qualitative information is available as to what precisely is being measured, what creates the putative functional short leg, how stable it might be, how it may be distinguished from an anatomical short leg, or what pathological significance a functional short leg may have.

Leg checking as triaxial assessment

Neither outright rejection nor uncritical faith in leg checking makes sense if leg checking is seen for what it is: a single component of what could be a full-fledged, bilateral determination of non-weight bearing foot posture. The foot, like any other segment of the body, is capable of deviating from a neutral postural position (however defined) in any of six degrees of freedom: three of translation and three of rotation. The conventional leg checker, in focusing on Y-axis "shortening" of the leg as evidenced by foot position, mostly ignores the other five degrees of freedom, to the point that he usually regards their variations as mere noise confounding the signal. Examples: "Correct for any inversion or eversion of the feet (can change listing)" (Thompson, 1984); "Remove inversion (supination) and plantar flexion" (Fuhr, 1997). Leg check skeptics, on the other hand, would toss out the baby with the bath water, since non-weight bearing foot postural assessment may be an important clue as to the function of the lumbopelvis and spine, all being part of the same kinematic chain.

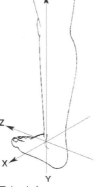

Triaxial perspective on foot asymmetry

Of the three possible translatory motions, a moment's reflection confirms that only longitudinal displacement of the foot on the Y-axis—the traditional functional short leg—seems clinically realistic, at least in the absence of ankle or foot fracture-dislocations. In that case, the short leg is not locally explained, but rather results from the relatively cephalad position of the entire lower extremity.

---

[1] Friberg O. Leg length inequality and low back pain. Clinical Biomechanics 1987;2:211-219.

All three rotational motions occur: X-axis dorsiflexion/plantarflexion, Z-axis inversion/eversion, and Y-axis internal/external rotation, or "foot flare." This foot flare is partly local, involving the subtalar joint, and partly the result of external hip rotation. Summarizing: the feet enjoy 4 degrees of freedom, two (shortening and flaring) involving at least in part the entire lower extremity, and two (dorsiflexion/plantarflexion and inversion/eversion) involving the foot and ankle alone.

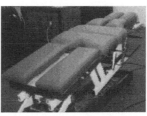
Friction-reduced table

To investigate unloaded non-weight bearing foot posture, model the leg checking procedure, and develop a triaxial measuring system, we constructed two novel devices: first, a friction-reduced table to measure Y-axis translatory components, and second, a triaxial inclinometric shoe to measure foot rotations.

We chose to model prone rather than supine leg checking, not only because it proved technically easier to do so, but because we believe prone leg checking to be more common in clinical practice. Work to date has centered primarily on modeling Y-axis translation on the table, and only recently has emphasized the assessment of rotational asymmetries

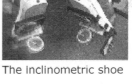
The Inclinometric shoe

using the inclinometric shoe. The full story of what we did and why will have to be told in some other time and place.

Traditional leg check theory inadequate

The prone leg check is ubiquitous among chiropractors. It has become axiomatic that the short leg side is pathognomonic of a PI ilium, the most typical explanation being that the hip would be drawn up by the posterior innominate rotation. As we have seen, this explanation depends on the erroneous belief that the-axis for the innominate rotation is located posterior to the hip joint, perhaps at the sacroiliac joint. It therefore follows that the usual explanation that has been offered to explain the short leg on the PI side must be wrong. It should be noted that apart from the inadequacy of a theory of the short leg that requires the symphysis pubis of the average patient to be dislocated, the traditional leg check model does not embrace the triaxial rotations (discussed and interpreted below).

Allegedly, as the innominate rotates posteriorly, the acetabulum swings superiorly. *What's wrong with this picture?*

The pelvic cleavage model, which designates a symphysis pubis-axis, swings the hip *inferiorly* and produces a physiological lengthening of the leg. As a matter of fact, *barring other influences,* one would expect to detect a physiological long leg in the prone leg check! The hip that is brought posterior and inferior in the weight bearing position would be expected to result in a more distally located knee and ankle joint in the prone position. Please note that this line of reasoning assumes "barring other influences" – and yet there are other influences. In other words, don't worry, the PI ilium does not result in a physiological long leg! Let us now explore these other influences, and in so doing save the time-honored proposition that the physiological short leg announces the side of the PI ilium.

Posterior torsion "lengthens" leg, although offset by other forces that result in functional short leg. (Fig. Hildebrandt, p.117)

A neo-classical leg check model

We must now elaborate an alternative model of what is detected by leg checking, and draw out the clinical implications. This will involve not only the "short leg" – translation of one leg relative to the other on the Y-axis – but the triaxial rotation findings.

Functional short leg checking (Y-axis linear translation)

The following discussion is written from the perspective of the PI ilium, it being understood that a symmetric analysis could have been written from the perspective of the AS ilium, with more or less identical results. It is also written on the basis of an assumption that there is little or no discrepancy in the length of the legs, as assumption that will be relaxed later in a more complete analysis. Since the hip joint is located posterior and superior to the symphysis, it follows that the head of the femur is carried posteriorly and inferiorly on the side of the PI ilium in the state of pelvic cleavage. The hip, which in a neutral postural position is carried just anterior to the ankle, is now carried posterior with respect to it. The hip and knee may flex slightly to accommodate this carriage of the hip. The net result is that the pelvis is unleveled, with the pelvic crest and ischium both lowered on the side of the PI ilium.

The paradox of the hypertonic, weak muscle

The sacral base is carried inferior on the side of the lowered innominate bone, resulting in an ipsilateral convex curvature of the lumbar spine. This creates some significant asymmetries in muscle length, tonus, and function. The ipsilateral trunk muscles, quadratus lumborum and sacrospinalis, will exist in a state of "stretch weakness"[2] whereas their contralateral counterparts will be in a state of "adaptative shortening." The ipsilateral thigh abductors (gluteus medius, tensor fascia lata) are found to be shortened, in a state of "postural abduction," whereas the contralateral thigh abductors are stretched, in a state of "postural adduction."

As chiropractors like Dr. Hugh Logan[3] have noted, the stretched muscles will exhibit a palpable hypertonicity. It is as thought they were "trying" to correct the postural imbalance - the sacrospinalis muscles want to hoist up the lowered sacral base, and the quadratus lumborum "wants to" raise the lowered innominate bone. This hypertonicity is, obviously, futile. Paradoxically, these hypertonic muscles will test weak on manual muscle testing, because a muscle which functions in a state of constant hypertonicity develops impaired function. "With continued, nonphysiological stimulatory impulses and the presence of permanently increased tonus, degenerative changes appear, resulting in the damage of the muscle fibers."

Anti-gravitational futility, recumbent success

The sacrospinalis and quadratus lumborum muscles are hypertonic on the PI ilium side, but futile in their anti-gravitational attempt to pull up the pelvis and the sacral base by their bootstraps, in the standing position. However, this futility becomes triumphant as soon as the patient is placed in the prone position. These muscles are no longer trying to raise the pelvis against gravity, but only against the resistance afforded by the *friction of the table* exerted upon the recumbent patient. (We will have more to say about this friction below.) As a general rule, the muscles succeed. The pelvis and lower extremity are indeed made more proximate to the rib cage on the side of the PI ilium. The hip, knee, and ankle are drawn up, accounting for the physiological short leg phenomenon. In fact, they are drawn up to a greater extent than the innominate rotation lowers these structures, as described above.

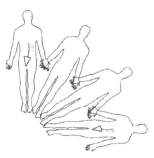

Muscles that are hypertonic but futile weight-bearing, become competent in a recumbent position.

---

[2] Kendall HO, Kendall FP, Wadsworth GE. Muscle testing and function. 2nd ed. Baltimore, MD: Williams & Wilkins; 1971.

[3] Logan HB. Textbook of Logan Basic Methods. St. Louis, Missouri: unknown; 1950.

Reversed muscle origin and insertion

These considerations explain a result that has been noted by many chiropractors. The PSIS is lowered on the PI side in the standing position, and yet it is elevated in the prone position. This apparent contradiction is fully explained by the fact that the hypertonic quadratus lumborum and sacrospinalis muscles are futile in the standing position and yet competent in the prone position. It's simply that the origin and insertions are reversed. In the standing position, the pelvis and sacrum become the fixed point or origin for the action of these muscles, which create by their contraction a lateral deviation of the spine; in the prone position, the trunk becomes the fixed position for these muscles, which wind up producing an elevation of the lower extremity. To use alternative terminology, it might be said that weight-bearing eccentric contraction yields to non-weight-bearing concentric contraction.

Clinical corollaries

There are a few simple procedures that may confirm this analysis. Measurement of the distance from the twelfth rib to the iliac crest will demonstrate approximation on the PI ilium side, a hoisting up of the lower extremity. Muscle relaxation techniques applied to the ipsilateral posterior trunk muscles may diminish or abolish the physiological short leg.

Gravity exerts a compressive force upon the spine that amplifies the postural distortions that would exist in a weightless condition, a condition in which the only compressive forces would be those introduced by the tonic contractions of the spinal musculature itself. Although the amplifying influence of gravity is lost in going from the weight-bearing to the prone position, and with it some of the diagnostic information, the examiner can still turn up the volume on the short leg detection system by tricking the body into thinking itself upright. He or she does this by exerting *a little* pressure on the feet. This manner of performing the leg check may increase observed leg length discrepancy.

The foot is invested with a multitude of proprioceptive structures that report directly to the postural control centers of the brain when the body is and when it is not in alignment with the earth's gravitational field. Cephalad pressure on the feet - evenly applied, of course - could stimulate the postural muscles to assume a state of tonicity in the prone position that would normally only be assumed in the standing position, thus increasing the observed amount of functional leg length inequality. (The vestibular apparatus would, of course, be generating contrary output to the brain).

On the other hand, *if more than a little pressure is applied*, an entirely different effect is introduced into the leg check, and indeed, an entirely different type of leg check is being performed. We call this type of leg check, in which enough cephalad force may be introduced to move the entire table, depending on what material covers the floor, the *compressive leg check*. This is certainly worth its own paragraph.

Compressive leg checking

The doctor applies very significant pressure to both legs, leaning forward into the leg check so that the patient may move cephalad on the table, and/or the table on the floor, depending on the relative degrees of friction at the patient-table and table-floor interfaces. We believe, although we have not yet proven the point, that any difference created in distal foot positions to reflect *structural* leg length inequality (LLI), in stark contrast to *functional* leg length inequality. We further believe that this type of maximum compression on the legs temporarily abolishes functional LLI. (There is also the possibility that there may be some sort of inherently enhanced joint compressibility on the PI side, which side in the opinion of many authors is subjected to increased rates of degenerative changes in the ankle, knee, and hip.) Obviously, we are not unaware that the gold standard for identifying and measuring structural leg length inequality is x-ray based, nor are we unaware of the various tape measure methods that have been described. However, the difficulty of obtaining such specialized x-rays and the inadequacy of the tape measure methods have led us to develop this compressive leg checking method.

Compressive leg checking enables us to truly understand the relationship between the leg check findings and other, principally lumbopelvic, findings. This pressure on the legs may increase, destroy, or reverse baseline LLI, although we are not in a position to explain all this until the next chapter, which ties together the various streams of information coming from the comprehensive examination of the lumbopelvis. Right now we had best emphasize the assessment methodology.

"Triaxial foot" leg checking: end-range rotations

In previous editions of this book I called a certain cluster of asymmetries in end-range passive foot movements the "sign of the PI foot." (Of course the foot was never really "PI". I was talking about a cluster of findings on the side of the PI ilium: functional short leg, external rotation, and inversion.) I used to say

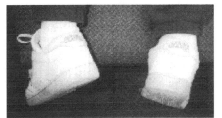

The triaxial (formerly "PI") foot.

that among the 3 possible rotations, although I was certain about inversion-eversion, and internal-external rotation, I was not sure about plantar and dorsiflexion, but that I thought plantarflexion tended to covary. (I also discussed, in this context, the covariance of accelerated wearing down of the posterolateral portion of the shoe.) Although the cluster could usually be seen on the prone patient with the feet untouched, I claimed the signs were usually more obvious at the end-point of passive ROM.

Having now had the opportunity to conduct my own (partially published) research on the matter, I am now able to refine the leg checking methodology previously described. The "PI foot" is now called "the triaxial foot," and I am reasonably certain that it corresponds to the side of the *lower hip* in the standing position. Since the hip may be carried inferiorly for at least two reasons, these being (1) anatomic LLI and (2) pelvic torsion, the term "PI foot" was too restrictive. Summarizing, the triaxial foot shows increased plantarflexion, inversion, and external rotation, and tends to occur on the side of the low hip. Next, we offer an explanation for each of the elements of the triaxial foot cluster.

Before doing so, let us be clear that there is not much of a diagnostic role left in all this for triaxial or conventional short leg determination.

External rotation

The external rotation about the y-axis is caused by the long term consequences of chronic piriformis

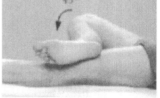

Most foot flare results from external hip rotation.

hyperactivity, initiated by an attempt to maintain postural homeostasis, given

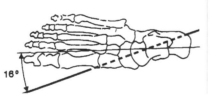

16°

Movement at subtalar joint contributes to appearance of foot flare

the lowering of the sacral base on the side of the posterior-inferior-medial ilium. This externally rotates the hip and gives rise to external foot rotation, often termed "foot flare" in chiropractic. Moreover, there is additive subtalar joint rotation; it seems that perhaps 2/3 of the foot flare comes from the external hip rotation, and other 1/3 is intrinsic to the foot.

Inversion

The increased inversion about the z-axis is caused by

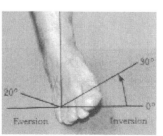

Inversion of the foot.

tibialis anterior hyperactivity, sustained as part of an unconscious attempt to maintain the integrity of the medial arch in walking and in standing. Indeed, this increased tone results in a groove in the navicular bone in the path of the insertion of the tibialis posterior muscle, according to the evidence on surgery for patients with tarsal tunnel syndrome related to pronation. There may be a contribution from tibialis posterior, which is also an invertor of the foot and exhibits increased tone due to the associated pronation.

It may seem paradoxical that the foot is relatively inverted (like supination) on the side of the posteriorly cleaved innominate bone. There is no inconsistency between this finding and the fact that the standing patient exhibits eversion (like pronation) of this same foot. During ambulation the neuromuscular control system attempts to compensate for the decreased height of the longitudinal arch by over-activating the tibialis anterior, which raises the arch and supinates the foot. This hyperactivity of the tibialis anterior may be so marked that it wears out a groove in the anterior medial plantar portion of the navicular bone, in the line of its tendon. "Apparently the bone effects were caused by long continued over activity of the tibialis anticus muscle tendon unit. This was the result of a maintained unconscious effort on the part of the patient to lift up the inner border of the foot in walking or standing." [4]

Whether or not these muscles are able to favorably effect the dynamic function of the foot in locomotion, in the standing position they are futile: the foot is pronated. Nonetheless, in the prone position the hypertonic contracture of the tibialis anterior is effective and the foot is inverted.

Plantar flexion

The increased plantarflexion about the X-axis is of less obvious origin. Perhaps it has to do with an unconscious effort to remain on the toes during walking, as if to compensate for the pelvic inferiority on that side of the body. This would increased the tone and activity of the gastrocnemius-soleus group. Or perhaps there is increased tone of tibialis posterior, a plantarflexion, attempting to maintain the integrity of the arch of the foot. It would be sharing that proclivity with tibialis anterior, a dorsiflexion, and would presumably overwhelm the dorsiflexing action of tibialis anterior.

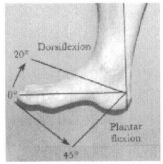

---

[4] Kopell, Thompson. Peripheral Entrapment Neuropathies.

Assessment of sitting-standing pelvic landmarks for anatomical LLI

When I described this test in a JACA artice ((Cooperstein, R. (2006). "Assessment of sitting-standing pelvic landmarks for anatomical LLI: Or Darwin's finches and leg checking." JACA 43(2): 12-14.)) I thought it was an original contribution. I now know better, having found it described by Bourdillon (Bourdillon, J. and E. Day (1987). Spinal Manipulation. Over Wallop, New Hamphsire, England, BAS Printers, Limited).

I am going to describe what I believe to be a novel visual test for anatomical leg length inequality (LLI). I had wanted to publish something on this test for some time, but desisted from doing so, for fear readers would find the description unconvincing in the absence of solid data and statistical analysis.

But then I got to thinking about Darwin's [darwin photo from powerpoint] trip to the Galapagos, and his famous finches. [finch illustration, in powerpoint) In *The Voyage of the* Beagle, Darwin wrote: "In the thirteen species of ground-finches, a nearly perfect gradation may be traced from a beak extraordinarily thick to one so fine that it may be compared with that of a warbler. I very much suspect that certain members of the series are confined to different islands."

It's a good thing Charles Darwin did not have to report his results at a chiropractic research conference, because a litany of audience members would have come to the microphone, demanding to know the following: the interexaminer reliability of counting finch species, and the operational definition of a finch as distinguished from a warbler. Someone else would have asked him if the observer who characterized the beaks had been adequately blinded from knowing upon which island the finches had been found. Darwin might have been so crushed he would never have gone on to write *The Origin of Species*. Well, if *he* was able to get away with publishing unblinded, perhaps preliminary data, then so should I. If you, the reader, are interested in LLI read on. If you are not interested in mere observation, albeit informed by basic science considerations and clinical experience, then this article may not be for you.

The most challenging problem in measuring the legs (short of a scanogram x-ray) is that there is no place to put the proximal end of the tape measure or other measuring apparatus. The distal end of the tape measure can be placed on a malleolus, but alas, there is no way to place the proximal end of the tape measure on or even near the femoral head. In lieu of that, investigators and clinicians have been placing the proximal end of the measure at the ASISs, the umbilicus, or the greater trochanters, with predictably poor interexaminer reliability and relatively unflattering concordance with scanogram x-ray – at least at the level of precision, say a few millimeters, that chiropractic clinicians would consider relevant.

Such measurement problems are far from insurmountable. Consider what it takes to measure the weight of a squealing toddler. Although there is no way to place the child on a floor-mounted scale, all we have to do is measure the weight of mom with and without the toddler in her arms. Thus, we can accomplish an indirect and yet very accurate measure of the toddler's weight. As an alternative, we could completely submerge little Johnny in a plastic tub filled to the brim with water (not for long!), and catch the overflow in yet another larger tub Then, measuring the volume of displaced water, and knowing that one liter of water weighs one kilogram, we would know his weight.

I am now in a position to describe an analogous indirect way to detect anatomical LLI. First, we locate the bilateral positions of a pelvic landmark, such as the PSISs (1), in the seated position. They may be on the same horizontal line, or there may be a height difference between the left and right sides. Then, being very careful to keep the palpating fingers in place, we have the subject stand. The landmarks are assessed once again. If the legs are indeed the same length, then the seated and standing landmarks should maintain their spatial relationship, remaining either on a horizontal line or showing the same difference as they did seated. If there is a difference between the seating and standing landmark positions (one might say, a delta between the seated-standing deltas), then there is likely to be leg length inequality.

In an unblinded study, the results of this sitting-standing indirect test for anatomic LLI was highly correlated with the results of compressive leg checking (3, 4), another procedure though to detect anatomic LLI, at about the 80% level of agreement. Subsequent refinements have led to even greater concordance of the two leg checking procedures, both at the college where I teach and in my private practice setting. I have not published anything on this, because I am both the PSIS palpator and the compressive leg checker, there having been no attempt at blinding. I assumed, and probably correctly so, that this preliminary observation would not be very convincing to some readers, even though the model at least generates testable hypotheses. I have since rethought the matter and decided to submit these initial observations for publication without further delay, although at the reader's own risk.

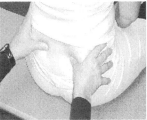

Palpating the pelvis for pelvic torsion

After all, initial observations may ultimately be proven wrong. Ironically, about one hour before beginning work on this article, while trying to make sense of some data gathered more rigorously in another study, I came across literature suggesting one of the more cherished rules for locating spinal landmarks is very, very questionable. Dr. Haneline (also at Palmer West) and I had performed a study that assumed, in its methodology, that the inferior tip of the scapula accurately locates the T7 spinous process. Careful data analysis suggested either we were inaccurate palpators, or that the rule simply didn't work. I am pleased to report that it was the rule, no doubt an unstudied observation that just kept getting published and taken for granted as such, that seems wrong. We are currently preparing a manuscript.

Nothing in life is risk-free. Keeping personal observations to oneself, for fear of publishing prematurely, may result in a related theory, potentially important, from ever seeing the light of day. It turns out that Charles Darwin was not the only naturalist to evolve a theory of natural selection. While he fiddled around for 20 years collecting and reconsidering his data, his contemporary Alfred Wallace came up with about the same theory, after having investigated much less and taken much less time. In one of the more memorable and commendable events in the history of science, they acknowledged each other's independent contributions and decided to publish the initial paper in collaboration: "The gentlemen having, independently and unknown to one another, conceived the same very ingenious theory to account for the appearance and perpetuation of varieties and of specific forms on our planet, and both fairly claim the merit of being original thinkers in this important line of inquiry" (Published in *Journal of the Proceedings of the Linnean Society*, Zoology 3: 45-62. 20 Aug 1858.) It is a lot easier to be like Wallace than like Darwin, when you teach as many courses as I do, while trying to do see patients and have a private life!

Notes for discussion of sitting-standing indirect test for aLLI

1. Cooperstein R. Palpating the pelvis for torsion. J Am Chiropractic Assoc 2004;41(9):48-50.
2. Cooperstein R, Lisi A. Pelvic torsion: anatomical considerations, construct validity, and chiropractic examination procedures. Topics in Clinical Chiropractic 2000;7(3):38-49.
3. Cooperstein R, Morschhauser E, Lisi A. Cross-sectional validity of compressive leg checking in measuring artificially created leg length inequality. Journal of Chiropractic Medicine 2004;3(3):91-95.
4. Cooperstein R, Morschhauser E, Lisi A, Nick T. Validity of compressive leg checking in measuring artificial leg length inequality. J Manipulative Physiol Ther 2003;26(9):557-566.

The clinical significance of leg checking

We have seen how and why there is reason to expect a functional short leg on the side of an inferior hip (i.e., iliac crest) be it related to pelvic torsion or anatomical short leg. We have also described two novel forms of distal leg assessment: end-range triaxial foot examination, and compressive leg checking. Clinical implementation of leg check results is discussed in the next chapter.

9. Leg length related pelvic syndromes

Having gone over a multiplicity of examination procedures for the lumbopelvis, which included standing, sitting, supine and prone findings, we need to tease out for special attention a series of syndromes. Each of these has to do with how anatomical asymmetry of leg lengths relates to pelvic torsion. In addition to detailing the relationships, we need to understand how these in turn result in typical examination findings, principally PSIS locations and leg checks. There is a significant amount of research out there, including some done by myself, part of it published and part not. It would get in the way of the story to constantly refer back to various references, and explicitly state what is an experimental finding, what seems very plausible in view of anatomical and physiological explanations, and which elements of the story remain quite speculative. Please bear with me.

Standing and sitting PSIS positions

The position of the standing PSIS is determined by the additive impact of at least two

> PSIS height is a function of pelvic torsion and relative leg lengths. The rough equation may be drawn:
>
> ΔPSIS (torsion) + ΔPSIS (LLI) = ΔPSIS (standing)

variables: relative leg lengths, and pelvic torsion. Anatomic short leg and posterior torsion would lower the femoral head, whereas anatomic long leg and anterior torsion would raise the femoral head. These two influences may be of same or opposite sign. Of course, we couldn't have the foot go through the floor when the innominate rotates posteriorly, lowering the hip; nor could we have the patient hopping around on his opposite foot when the innominate rotates anteriorly, raising the hip. We presume that the hip and knee flex on the relatively posterior side, which accommodates the lowering of the acetabulum on the PI side, and prevents loss of continuity with the ground on the AS side. Hugh Logan, to his credit, described this hip and knee "flex," in his masterpiece, *Basic Technique*.

When the legs are equal in length, and there is no pelvic torsion, we would expect the standing PSISs to be on a horizontal line. The exception would be in the case of innominate structural asymmetry, although I am unaware of data on how frequently this occurs.

When there is a minor degree of anatomic short leg, say 3 mm or less, the innominate bone tends to rotate *posteriorly* on the short leg side, resulting in a greater amount of PSIS discrepancy. This could be called a "decompensated" anatomic LLI syndrome. This makes sense, given the axis for hemipelvic rotation through the symphysis pubis: as the acetabulum is lowered due to the short leg, the innominate bone is likely to rock

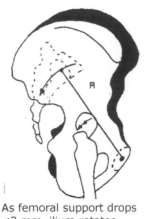

As femoral support drops <3 mm, ilium rotates posteriorward.

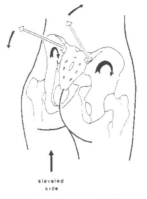

As femoral support drops <3 mm, ilium rotates anteriorward to compensate.

posteriorly, in addition to the lateral tilting of the entire pelvis that would occur. Thus, one would expect to find a PI ilium on the side of the anatomic short leg. Lateral full pelvic tilting and ipsilateral posterior hemipelvic rotation produce an additive lowering of the PSIS in the standing position.

When there is a more marked degree of anatomic short leg, say 3 mm or more, the innominate bone tends to rotate anteriorly, as the result of compensatory muscle tone asymmetries. Thus, one would expect to find an AS ilium on the side of the anatomic short leg. Innate intelligence (the unconscious neuromusculoskeletal control mechanism, if you prefer) appears willing to put up with small amounts of anatomic LLI, allowing the hemipelvis to slip into some degree of posterior torsion. This happens to be about the amount of LLI investigators have found just beneath the amount that predicts low back pain, interestingly enough. Innate intelligence seems to insist upon an opposite and compensatory *anterior* hemipelvic rotation when the amount of LLI is likely to lead to low back pain.

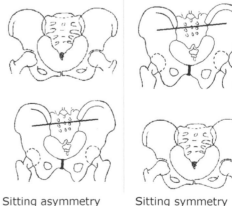

Sitting asymmetry (below) associated with standing symmetry (above), suggesting offsetting torsion and LLI.

Sitting symmetry (below) associated with standing asymmetry (above) suggests anatomic LLI.

In the sitting position, with LLI taken out of the picture for obvious reasons, we presume any visible unleveling of the PSISs to be the result of pelvic torsion. This torsion could be primary, meaning unrelated to anatomic LLI, or secondary, compensatory to anatomic LLI. The illustration to the near right depicts a patient with a right anatomical LLI, compensated by right AS, left PI pelvic torsion. This levels the PSISs in the standing position. (Indeed, it is a mistake to assume that level PSISs in the standing position argue against anatomic leg length discrepancy, as is commonly done.)

The patient depicted in the far right illustration does not have any pelvic torsion, given the sitting finding that the PSISs are even. On the other hand, the unleveling of the PSISs in the standing position suggests anatomic LLI, uncompensated by torsion. Thus, this may be termed an "uncompensated" LLI syndrome.

Sitting iliac crest evaluation

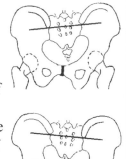

The examiner should compare the difference in iliac crest heights in the sitting position as compared with the standing position. It is intuitively obvious that with the legs taken out of the picture, by virtue of the subject being seated, anatomic leg length inequality cannot cause asymmetry in the location of the PSISs. There are data suggesting that congenital asymmetry of the innominate bones tends to be rather minimal, so that sitting pelvic asymmetry is better explained by subluxation than congenital factors. Under the assumption of left-right hemipelvic symmetry, and a further assumption that the doctor has not failed to notice a wallet or other object in one of the subject's rear pockets, then there is likely to be

Standing-sitting PSIS reversals suggest more complicates situations.

interinnominate torsion if the PSISs are not on a true horizontal. The low side, of course, reflects a relative posterior hemipelvic rotation and the high side a relative anterior rotation. True comprehension of the subject's overall lumbopelvic configuration requires juxtaposition of this information, such as the results of compressive and triaxial leg checking, and standing PSIS locations. That is described comprehensively below, at the end of this chapter.

In the meantime, if a significant differential in the standing position is reduced, disappears, or even reverses in going to a seated position, there is a strong suggestion that there is anatomical leg length inequality that is partially or fully offset, or even reversed by pelvic torsion, so that the pelvis may wind up level or even elevated on the side of the anatomic short leg.

Palpating the pelvis for torsion

Chiropractors, physical therapists, and osteopaths all seem fairly obsessed with the short leg syndrome, partly because asymmetry of the lower extremities is thought to have painful consequences for the patient, and partly because it is thought to have diagnostic significance. As someone who has spent many years studying the purported relation of leg length inequality (LLI) to pelvic torsion, it was not without a sense of chagrin that I have finally came to the conclusion that to make a mechanical diagnosis of the pelvis, it is usually better to examine the pelvis than, well, the feet (i.e., leg checking). This column develops my reasons for having come to this conclusion.

In chiropractic, leg checking is used in a number of circumstances:

- To assess the status of the atlanto-occipital joint;
- To look for evidence of anatomical LLI
- To serve as an outcome measure following provocative procedures (e.g., Derifield leg check (1), isolation testing (2), etc.)
- As an outcome measure to track the patient's short and long term response to chiropractic adjustive care.
- To identify pelvic torsion (3);

Anthony Lisi and I (3) coauthored a review article on pelvic torsion in which, among other topic areas covered, we described the various direct and indirect methods that have been claimed to detect pelvic torsion. These included radiographic, inclinometric, visual, palpatory, and reflex methods. Among the palpatory methods, some are direct, involving identification of pelvic anatomical landmarks, and others are indirect, such as pressure testing (2) and leg checking (4).

Although limitations of space prevent me from reviewing the advantages and disadvantages of these various methods for detecting pelvic torsion, let alone its clinical significance, at least let us assume it might be worth having a quick, low-tech, noninvasive method for identifying pelvic torsion from visit to visit. Since among the listed procedures leg checking more than any other assessment procedure fits that bill, we need to see if current models connecting leg check findings with LLI make sense. It is commonly believed that there is posterior innominate rotation on the side of a functional short leg, and relative anterior rotation on the opposite side.

One would assume that every leg checker, at some point in his or her career, conceives the thought, however transiently, that one leg appears shorter than the other simply *because it is*. Although the overall literature is somewhat equivocal, Friberg (5) using scanogram x-ray found that about half of asymptomatic research participants and about 75% of patients with low back pain exhibited LLI of 1/4" or more. Since things are sometimes just as simple as they seem, given the how common anatomic LLI appears to be, why start out by assuming that observed LLI results from subluxation in the pelvis, upper cervical area, or any other region of the body?

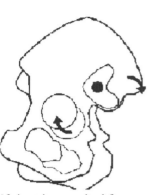

If short leg resulted from posterior rotation swinging up the hip, the front of the pelvis would dislocate.

Even if observed LLI were to result from innominate subluxation (i.e., were to constitute functional LLI), there are problems with the mechanism that is usually described. The most common explanation of the PI=short leg rule has a posterior swing of the innominate bone pulling the acetabulum, and therefore the lower extremity, cephalad (6, 7). This explanation can also be found in the physical therapy literature (8) and apparently in osteopathy (presentation by David Grimshaw, D.O., American Back Society, Las Vegas, Nevada, 1999).

This explanation requires the interinnominate axis of rotation to be posterior to the hip, perhaps through the sacroiliac joint. However, if the hip were indeed carried cephalad by this mechanism, then so would the pubic ramus, and by a much larger amount (Figure 1). In fact, a 6 mm short leg created in this way would luxate the symphysis pubis by causing a diastasis of around half an inch (9). For this reason, this explanation is not very appealing.

A more patient-friendly approach to explaining the association of posterior innominate rotation and the functional short leg invokes greater suprapelvic muscle tone on the side of posterior innominate rotation (4, 10, 11), as part of a postural reflex. Relative hypertonus of the quadratus lumborum and/or sacrospinalis muscles, although unable to elevate the hemipelvis in a standing patient, would elevate the lower extremity in a prone or supine patient, creating a "muscular short leg," as Schneider puts it (11).

But why bother *inferring* pelvic torsion from a leg check, whatever the purported connection, when a direct method could be used? It is intuitively obvious that rotation of one innominate bone anteriorly, while the other rotates relatively posterior, must change the position of the anterior and posterior iliac spines (ASISs and PSISs). Levangie {Levangie, 1999 #799}has used sitting PSIS unleveling as evidence of pelvic torsion.

Why sitting? In the standing position, unleveling of the PSISs reflects the additive effect of both anatomic LLI and pelvic torsion. In fact, anatomic LLI can result in pelvic torsion (12-15), making it especially difficult to tease out the separate contributions (anatomic short leg results in compensatory anterior innominate rotation). In the seated position, difference in structural leg length can not effect PSIS positions, leaving pelvic torsion as the infinitely better explanation of any observed PSIS asymmetry.

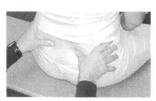

Seated PSIS palpation

Before jumping to the conclusion that seated PSIS asymmetry *must* reflect pelvic torsion, we still need to consider the possibility that congenital differences in innominate dimensions may account for observed PSIS asymmetry. Little was known about such hypothetical innominate asymmetry until fairly recently. Evidence from CT scanning (16) and also from direct measuring (17) tells the same story: congenital asymmetry of the innominate bones is minimal. Therefore, it is likely that seated PSIS asymmetry reflects pelvic subluxation rather than innominate dysplasia.

The examiner should palpate the PSISs of the seated patient in three positions: coming down toward them from above with the thumbs pressing firmly into the soft tissue, coming in from below with firm pressure, and finally right at the most posterior aspect of the PSISs. (See figure 2.) The examiner would have the most confidence in the exam findings when all 3 positions provide the same result. The inferior side, of course, reflects a relative posterior hemipelvic rotation and the superior side a relative anterior rotation. Which sacroiliac joint is to be adjusted, if not both, depends on additional clinical information – symptoms, orthopedic testing, postural evaluation, and reflex testing procedures.

The examiner will find it very interesting to observe what happens upon having the patient rise to the standing position with the thumbs still in place, and then sit again, thumbs still in place. Sitting asymmetry may disappear standing, and reappear while sitting; or vice versa. This sitting-standing procedure is very useful to demonstrate the existence of anatomical LLI.

Notes for this section on palpating for pelvic torsion

1.   Cooperstein R. The Derifield pelvic leg check: a kinesiological interpretation. Chir Tech 1991;3(2):60-65.
2.   Fuhr AW, Green JR. Activator Methods analytic technique. In: Chir Tech. St. Louis: Mosby; 1997. p. 92-110.
3.   Cooperstein R, Lisi A. Pelvic torsion: anatomical considerations, construct

validity, and chiropractic examination procedures. Topics in Clinical Chiropractic 2000;7(3):38-49.

4.   Cooperstein R. Integrated Chiropractic Technique: Chiropraxis. Oakland, CA: Self-published; 2000.

5.   Friberg O. Leg length inequality and low back pain. Clinical Biomechanics 1987;2:211-219.

6.   Gatterman MI. Chiropractic management of spine-related disorders. Baltimore MD: Williams & Wilkins; 1990.

7.   Bergmann T, Peterson DH, Lawrence DJ. Chiropractic Technique. New York, NY: Churchill Livingstone Inc.; 1994.

8.   Manheimer J, Lampe G. Clinical Transcutaneous Electrical Nerve Stimulation. Philadelphia: F. A. Davis Company; 1984.

9.   Cooperstein R. Functional leg length inequality: geometric analysis and an alternative muscular model. In: 8th Annual Conference on Research and Education; 1993; Monterey, California: Consortium for Chiropractic Research California Chiropractic Association; 1993. p. 202-203.

10.   Travell JG, Simons DG. Myofascial Pain and Dysfunction: The Trigger Point Manual. The Lower Extremities. Baltimore: Williams and Wilkins; 1992.

11.   Schneider M. The "muscular" short leg. American Journal of Clinical Chiropractic 1993;3(3):8.

12.   Beaudoin L, Zabjek KF, Leroux MA, Coillard C, Rivard CH. Acute systematic and variable postural adaptations induced by an orthopaedic shoe lift in control subjects. Eur Spine J 1999;8(1):40-5.

13.   Drerup B, Hierholzer E. Movement of the human pelvis and displacement of related anatomical landmarks on the body surface. J Biomech 1987;20(10):971-7.

14.   Young RS, Andrew PD, Cummings GS. Effect of simulating leg length inequality on pelvic torsion and trunk mobility. Gait Posture 2000;11(3):217-23.

15.   Cummings G, Scholz JP, Barnes K. The effect of imposed leg length difference on pelvic bone symmetry. Spine 1993;18(3):368-73.

16.   Badii M, Shin S, Torreggiani WC, Jankovic B, Gustafson P, Munk PL, et al. Pelvic Bone Asymmetry in 323 Study Participants Receiving Abdominal CT Scans. Spine 2003;28(12):1335-9.

17.   Thompson DM, Vrugtman R. Biometric comparison of the heights and widths of paired innominates. Journal of Chiropractic Education 2003;17(1):39-40.

Sitting leg check

It is possible to assess the relative position of the medial malleoli of a sitting patient. Although any difference observed may result from congenital or acquired asymmetry of tibial lengths, it is also plausible that a difference may reflect a difference in the tissue stiffness of the hamstring muscles. That is, the stiffer the tissue, the "shorter" the sitting leg will appear (the more raised off the examination table). I intend to investigate this phenomenon in the future, and so it is premature to suggest any one particular interpretation of sitting malleoli positions. Later on in this text, I provide a kinesiological interpretation of the prone Derifield pelvic leg check, the analytic engine of which depends on asymmetry of anterior thigh tissue stiffness. Suffice it to say that asymmetry of posterior tissue stiffness is a phenomenon also worthy of interpretation, in due time.

PSIS locations as related to leg checks

The triaxial foot identifies the side of the standing low hip, whether due to anatomic LLI, pelvic torsion, or any combination thereof. There may be a small LLI with additive posterior innominate rotation, a larger degree of LLI with inadequate anterior innominate rotation, or primary pelvic torsion in the absence of LLI.

The compressive short leg identifies an anatomic short leg, and therefore allows us to differentiate between primary pelvic torsion and secondary pelvic torsion, related to LLI in a variety of patterns (see chart below).

The conventional functional short leg covaries with the triaxial foot, but there is a substantial possibility of confounding findings. With a small degree of anatomical LLI, we expect the functional short leg, triaxial foot, and compressive short leg to all be on the same side. With a larger degree of anatomical LLI, anterior pelvic rotation may level the hips or *even raise* the standing hip on the side of the structural short leg. When this latter situation occurs, we expect the compressive short leg to be opposite the functional short leg and the triaxial foot.

Since both seem to relate to a standing low hip, it is not obvious, what, if anything, would cause the functional short leg to not covary with the triaxial foot, irrespective of the compressive leg check findings. Nonetheless, we are hard-pressed to explain this finding, which we do see from time to time. (Primary muscle hypertonus opposite the side of posterior innominate rotation, secondary to trauma, herniated disk, etc?)

Examination protocol

We must obtain sitting and standing PSIS levels, and perform at least the compressive and triaxial leg checks; the conventional functional short leg determination seems at

Suggested sequence for relating leg checks and PSIS findings:

• standing postural assessment, including PSIS heights
• sitting PSIS assessment
• triaxial leg check
• compressive leg check

best redundant if a careful triaxial determination is accomplished, and at worst purely confusing when its result differs from the triaxial result. I suggest the following sequence: standing PSIS heights, sitting PSIS heights, prone triaxial leg check, and finally the prone compressive leg check.

Treatment implications

First, let us state there are no data on how best to treat pelvic torsion, let alone torsional syndromes related to anatomical LLI. There is nothing unusual about this lack of data, there being very little information in general about which adjustive strategies work best for specific low back conditions. As always, we note that lack of evidence is certainly not equivalent to evidence of lack. That stated, we think it appropriate to offer a few suggestions related to torsion syndromes.

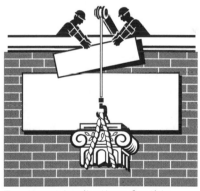

As a general rule, provided the patient is symptomatic, it is *a priori* reasonable to adjust so as to reduce the torsional state, whether it amounts to anterior or posterior rotation on the side of an anatomic LLI, or is a primary hemipelvic torsion. Nonetheless, the syndrome of "compensated" LLI, with anterior rotation, is more treacherous, and

Treatment implications for this approach are under construction.

should be treated with increased "respect." Less force, more specificity, more prudence.

The syndrome of decompensated LLI, with posterior rotation on the LLI side, resembles (but is not identical to) Logan's Basic Distortion: rotatory scoliosis, convex on the side of the low sacrum, and the posteriorly rotated innominate bone. Here, we are more comfortable applying more general forces, utilizing rotational vectors, producing multiple cavitation events. (We are in the zone of the $50.00 roll, as described in one of the chapters below.) The case of the primary PI reduces to the same set of considerations, and there is little to worry about.

With a significant degree of anatomic LLI, consideration must be given to introducing a heel lift, but that is pretty much beyond the scope of this text. Suffice it to say that it is not uncommon to find that a patient with appreciable LLI may have low back and /or more remote symptoms that do not adequately ameliorate with adjustive care. Whether we opine that this patient's adjustments are not "holding" (whatever that means), or offer up some other explanation for the problem, we should consider the use of heel lifts or shoe modifications of some sort.

I used to think that pelvic torsion was not very reducible through adjustive care, and there is some evidence that thrusts of certain types do not ameliorate it. However, careful pre-post inspection of patients has led me to believe that there is some degree of reduction, although often it has not been maintained by the time of the next office visit.

Derifield pelvic leg check

As is described in more detail in the next chapter entitled "The Derifield Pelvic Leg Check," there is reason to believe that the D+ finding points toward primacy of the posteriorly-rotated innominate side, whereas the D- finding implicates the relatively anteriorly-rotated innominate side. Admittedly, this is an awfully arbitrary and simplistic adage, smacking of rule-ism. Nevertheless, I must confess to using it, at least as an element in a multivariate decision-making process.

The preceding chapter described the rationale and procedure for leg checking, prematurely perhaps, since this is rightfully part of the prone examination of the subject; but it seemed appropriate to take care of this very traditional and ubiquitous chiropractic examination procedure right out of the gate, in its own chapter. That stated, we will recapitulate a few of the conclusions that were drawn.

Physiological (functional) shortening of the leg occurs on the side of the inferior hemipelvis, whether due to pelvic torsion or anatomic LLI. (In the later case, functional LLI is additive to the anatomic LLI). The magnitude of this inequality may be somewhat increased if the examiner exerts a little (less than the amount of pressure used in compressive leg checking, described below) cephalad pressure on the feet. Hypothetically, this "tricks" the kinesthetic proprioceptors of the foot into supposing that the body is in the weight-bearing position, which in turn will cause the brain to activate the anti-gravity muscles. (The vestibular apparatus, of course, would be sending contrary information.) This would increase the hypertonicity of the quadratus lumborum muscle and sacrospinalis muscles enough to slightly draw up the leg, enough to increase the observed leg length inequality.

Triaxial foot findings on side of the weight-bearing inferior hemipelvis: increased end-range passive plantarflexion, inversion, and external rotation (abduction). The triaxial findings are more consistent than simple functional short leg determination, although they covary. Therefore, we propose that the triaxial check in essence replace the more traditional functional short leg determination, pending more research. The triaxial foot usually occurs on PI side, whether the legs are structurally even or not. With anatomical LLI, the triaxial foot supplements posterior innominate rotation in leveling the sacral base on the long leg side. Thus, the triaxial foot occurs on the side of the prone long leg, as checked conventionally. When there is no anatomic LLI, the triaxial foot occurs on the side of the prone short leg, conventionally checked, as part of the primary PI ilium syndrome. Flow charts following the next chapter make this more clear.

Compressive leg check shows asymmetry of distal leg positions when there is congenital or acquired anatomical leg length inequality. This test requires much more force than the mild compression described above under "physiological" (or functional) short leg. It is not uncommon to see mild asymmetry increase under mild pressure, and then become obliterated or even reversed under higher compression. This suggests that sometimes there may be a functional short leg on the side of an anatomical long leg, which amounts to saying that the torsional effect on innominate height overwhelms the leg length delta effect. For example, a right anatomic short leg is compensated by right anterior rotation, that is so effective that the standing subject has a high iliac crest on the right, the side of the short leg.

Appendix: structural LLI protocol

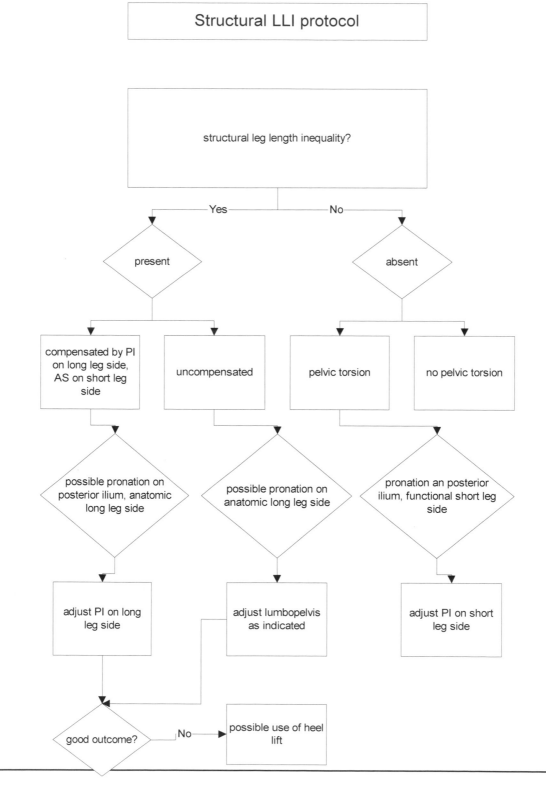

10. The Derifield pelvic leg check: A kinesiological interpretation

We have already extensively discussed chiropractic leg checking, both conventional functional short leg determination and more novel forms under development (triaxial, compressive). The *Derifield leg check* is a more detailed protocol, worthy of its own standalone chapter. The bulk of this chapter is based on work previously published in the journal *Chiropractic Technique*[1]

Cervical and pelvic components of the Derifield leg check

First, I have seen the spelling of this leg check rendered as both "Derifield" and "Derefield," but believe the former spelling more authoritative. This decidedly "cookbook" procedure is performed by a variety of technique adherents, including practitioners of Activator Methods, Thompson Technique, and Pierce-Stillwagon Technique; and is also routinely performed by many clinicians who would characterize themselves as Diversified or eclectic practitioners. Interpretations abound as to the significance of the cervical and pelvic components.

In the cervical portion of the Derifield leg check, the prone patient actively rotates his or her head to both the left and right sides, to see if any baseline difference in distal leg positions is altered. In my own research involving the friction-reduced table (table mentioned in an earlier chapter) I was able to see such changes occur from time to time, usually a relative shortening on the side to which the head was turned.[2] I interpreted this to be a manifestation of the tonic neck reflex, a normal occurrence in adults (unlike, for example, pathological reflex such as Babinski), and thus see no basis at this time to find such changes indicative of subluxation (of anything). I reserve the right to change this opinion if and when I get an opportunity to continue this line of research, but for now, I do not perform the cervical component of the Derifield leg check.

---

[1] Cooperstein R. The Derifield pelvic leg check: a kinesiological interpretation. Chiropractic Technique 1991;3(2):60-65.

[2] Cooperstein R, Bricker D, Jansen R. Detection of absolute and relative left and right leg displacements as a function of head rotation: the advantages of using a friction-reduced multi-segmented table. In: Cleveland III C, Haldeman S, editors. Conference Proceedings of the Chiropractic Centennial Foundation; 1995; Washington, DC: Chiropractic Centennial Foundation; 1995. p. 323-324.

The pelvic portion of the Derifield leg check compares prone distal leg positions with the knees extended compared with when the knees are flexed to 90^0. There was a time when I could not imagine how this could determine anything other than a possible anatomical asymmetry of tibial lengths, where the shorter tibia would not hold the foot as high off the table when the knees are both at 90^0.

At this time I have come to a different conclusion, and now see asymmetry in flexed-knee foot heights to represent the *additive result* of possible tibial asymmetry and lower extremity soft tissue flexibility differences, as discussed below. The discussion below, for the most part, discounts the possible asymmetric tibial length contribution, not because there is any reason to think it insignificant, but because model building sometimes requires such simplifying assumptions, just to move forward at all. This model is data-free, but bears considerable concept validity. It also generates many testable hypotheses, and someday I hope to do just that, test them. That will be the time to work tibial asymmetry in the larger scheme of things. In the meantime, as the reader will see, the so-called "paper sign," proposed below as an orthopedic test that correlates with the other Derifield findings, should permit the distinction of the case of tibial asymmetry from that of lower extremity soft tissue differences. But I fear I am getting ahead of myself . . .

Previous studies

The Derifield pelvic leg check (DPLC) purports to detect pelvic dysfunction, categorize its type, and indicate the clinical means by which it can be corrected. In the case of a Positive Derifield (D+), the physiological short leg in position 1 (knees extended, prone position) evens up with or becomes longer than the other in position 2 (patient's legs flexed to approximately 90 degrees). In the case of Derifield Negative (D-), the short leg in position 1 stays short or appears even shorter in position 2. [1]

Researchers have made some headway in assessing the inter-examiner reliability of the DPLC [2,3], but its biomechanical interpretation remains obscure. Frogley claims that the DPLC distinguishes sacral from ilium subluxation, but offers no particular rationale for his supposition [4]. Although Thompson presents no biomechanical explanation of D+, we infer from the correctional strategy he employs that he considers D+ to indicate a "garden variety" PI ilium, whereas D- is explicitly said to involve hamstring tension and sacral inferiority [5]. In Activator Technique, D+ would indicate lumbar body rotation toward the short leg side, and D- lumbar body rotation away from the short leg side [6]. Most field practitioners employing the DPLC would probably agree that the DPLC detects in some way "spinal stress" or "muscle contractures" related to subluxation.

Although these various interpretations of the DPLC are not necessarily inconsistent with one another, none of them is detailed enough to qualify as a legitimate explanation. There is no basis for allowing a rational discrimination among their validities. Even granted a respectable degree of reliability, an assessment tool cannot be properly used unless it 1) defines concretely what entity is being assessed; 2) explains how the tool assesses the entity. The failure of the DPLC on this level has jeopardized its status, and rightfully so, among both investigators and clinicians [7].

Nonetheless, the chiropractic profession should not reject empirically developed diagnostic procedures simply because they have not been adequately explained. Although we must not hesitate to militantly abandon diagnostic tools that are explicitly anti-anatomical or physiologically impossible, we should with equal militancy erect wherever possible plausible explanations that generate testable hypotheses. According to the economist Milton Friedman, "The only relevant test of the validity of a hypothesis is comparison of its predictions with experience" [8]. What follows is just such an analysis of the Derifield leg check.

The trigonometry of pelvic syndrome

It is difficult to see why legs that are uneven in the knees-extended position would not even out in the knees-flexed position. After all, it would seem that no matter what event proximal to the lower extremity had drawn one leg up in position 1, it

Fig. 1. The left hip, knee, and foot are drawn up uniformly by supra-pelvic muscle contractures. Leg-length inequality is created in position II because one knee is more cephalad when the feet are approximated in position II.

would be removed from the picture in position 2. In other words, if the tibias are of equal length, then it would be reasonable to expect them to appear that way!

As a case in point, let us suppose that by some physiological mechanism, such as the extensor muscle contractures that are invoked by Thompson [9], that one hip joint is pulled upward relative to the other in the prone position. Then the knee is drawn up and so is the foot, all on the same side. We still fully expect, all other things being equal, the feet to even up when the knees are flexed. [The reader is invited to use his arms as surrogate legs: with arms outstretched and elbows extended, give yourself a one inch short "leg." Now, flex your "knees" so that your

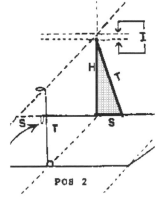

Fig. 1a. Detail from fig. 1, where shaded triangle indicates how the Pythagorean theorem may be applied to calculate "I"

pisiforms are approximated. The "feet" even up for obvious reasons.]

An astute observer might have noticed that if a hip and knee are drawn up by muscle contractures and in this manner account for the prone short leg, that when the malleoli are approximated in the flexed positions the knees cannot geometrically entertain the same degrees of flexion. This could in principle account for a short leg either staying short or crossing over to become the long leg in position 2, depending on which leg is brought closer to 90^0. Unfortunately, the numbers are simply not there. Simple trigonometry shows that this can explain only about 1/100 inch of apparent leg length inequality in the flexed position (figures 1 and 1a). Relatively trivial mathematical checks such as this enable us to avoid attributing quantitative and therefore clinical significance to marginal mechanical effects such as these.

Kinesiological hypotheses

There are only two mechanisms that could explain how the legs could appear uneven in position 2, leaving aside the trivial possibility of examiner error [10]:

• The tibias are not anatomically equal in length. Given inequality, we would expect the short leg in position 1 to remain the short leg in position 2. In this situation the Derifield leg check simply detects anatomical leg length inequality.

• When the knees are passively flexed, the thigh is elevated from the table for some reason, and more so on one side than the other.

In the case of the second mechanism, we might suppose that the patellofemoral joint is involved: increased quadriceps tonus could interfere with the descent of the patella as the knee flexed, so that the thigh would rest at least to some degree on the patella. This would result in an elevation of the foot on this side. In reality, although there is a condition called patella alta [11] in which the patella is fixated superiorly, it is not especially common, and certainly has an incidence rate considerably less than what has been reported for Pelvic Syndrome. As an alternative hypothesis, we might suppose that as the knees are passively flexed, increased quadriceps tonus on one side could exert tension upon the patellofemoral ligament and in this manner compress the joint space between flexed tibia and the femur upon which it is erected. Perhaps, but it is not plausible to presume that enough diminution of joint space could occur in this manner to account for the leg length alterations that clinicians are claiming to have observed.

Let us now consider another mechanism that is more likely to account for typical

DPLC findings. We first assume quadriceps hypertonicity (etiology unknown) on one or the other leg. We know that a hypertonic muscle may be made to relax by employing either a rapidly applied stretch which provokes the Golgi tendon organ to reflexively inhibit muscle tone [12], or by a long duration stretch that permits a viscoelastic lengthening of the muscle [13]. However, we also know that a less accelerated and shorter duration stretch of a hypertonic muscle would be expected to result in an increase in muscle tone, by means of the static stretch reflex [14]. In other words, hypertonic muscles are in a constant state of irritation. Their initial response to a mild and brief static stretch is to become further irritated and increase their degree of hypertonicity [15].

This reflex stimulation increases the anteroposterior diameter of the quadriceps muscle, lifting the thigh slightly off the table and increasing the height of the leg. More precisely, this reflex stimulation diminishes the extent to which the quadriceps muscle belly is flattened against the table by its own weight in position 2. The magnitude of this effect is moreover directly related to the firmness of the table.

One would suppose that such an effect could occur on either the short or long leg side as assessed in position 1. If it were to occur on the short leg side, we would have accounted for a D+ finding - the short leg not only evens up (this evening alone is an automatic consequence of the anatomic equality of the tibias) but actually appears to become longer than the other leg. If, on the other hand, this effect were to occur on the long leg side, then the long leg remains long in position 2 (equivalent to the short leg remaining short), the D- finding.

We may summarize as follows:

• A short leg which evens up when flexed indicates anatomically equal tibias;

• A short leg which crosses over to become long in position 2 signifies an ipsilaterally hypertonic quadriceps (D+);

• A short leg which remains short indicates a contralaterally hypertonic quadriceps on the long leg side (D-).

A synthetic Derifield finding

It is not hard to put these hypotheses to an initial test. We wish to know if the state of contraction of the quadriceps can alter the observed leg length in

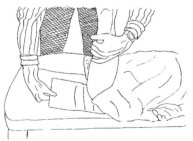

Fig 2. Paper sign identifies leg with more anterior thigh stiffness.

position 2. The prone patient in position 2 is asked to very mildly attempt to straighten a flexed knee against the examiner's resistance, while the latter observes the relative positions of the feet. It will be noted upon performing this test that the foot on the contracted side will rise, to an extent directly proportional to the magnitude of the patient's isometric effort. This constitutes a synthetic Derifield, either positive or negative depending on whether the contraction is induced on the short or the long leg side, respectively.

The paper sign

In order to prove that the mechanism has to do with the quadriceps exhibiting a reduced compressive force against the table, the examiner may place a piece of paper under both knees, about 3 inches in (figure 2). The examiner assesses how much force is required to pull the paper out from under the knee, and then repeats the procedure as the patient exerts mild quadriceps contraction. The paper is considerably easier to withdraw during the contraction. This confirms that the relatively increased AP quadriceps diameter has decreased the pressure of the thigh against the table, or perhaps its area of contact with the table. It is reasonable to suppose that this "paper sign" distinguishes differences in foot elevation due to asymmetry in tibial lengths (presumably, a negative paper sign) from those attributable to soft tissue asymmetry (positive paper sign).

Having synthesized a Derifield result under test conditions, the next task is to determine if a similar phenomenon exists under field conditions, among patients not asked to contract their quadriceps. A positive paper sign signifies a greater relative ease of withdrawal on one side compared to the other. It is best to draw a few horizontal lines on the paper to ascertain the extent to which it is placed underneath the distal thigh. It is usually necessary to try out a few degrees of insertion in order to identify where the maximal left/right distinction may be detected, owing to the fact that there is much variation among patients in the shape and soft tissue compliance of their thighs.

The paper sign represents an orthopedic test that confirms the existence of pelvic syndrome, indicates which is the involved side, and finally distinguishes D+ from D-. Our initial results have indicated a strong tendency for the paper sign to be positive on the short leg side in Derifield positive patients, and on the long leg sign in Derifield negative patients. The sign tends to become equivocal in cases where the short leg evens in position 2, in which case it is possible that both the right and left thigh flexors are hypertonic. Our results are more consistent when a firm table is used, insofar as a soft table tends to accommodate to both thighs and obliterates the sign.

It is also possible to evaluate what amounts to a reverse paper sign, in which we assess the degree to which a stiff piece of paper can be inserted under the prone knee. In a research setting, we developed a ruled transparency that allowed not only easy insertion but the determination of the distance of insertion.

D+ and D-: kinesiological implications

In a state of postural symmetry, the innominate bones are superimposable in the sagittal plane. Failing this, a state of pelvic torsion exists in which one innominate bone rotates anterior, superior, and laterally and the other posterior, inferior, and medially. We know from Hildebrandt's investigations that the axis for this pelvic torsion transects the symphysis transversely [16]. In common parlance chiropractors have traditionally used the listings "AS" and "PI" to describe this torsional effect. In the discussion below, following Hildebrandt, "posterior pelvic cleavage" is equivalent to a PI-IN ilium and "anterior pelvic cleavage" to an AS-EX ilium. The short leg in position 1 tends to occur on the side of posterior pelvic cleavage [17].

In D+, weak thigh flexors (primarily rectus femoris and sartorius) allow the short leg side innominate bone to subluxate posteriorly, inferiorly, and medially, resulting in posterior pelvic cleavage. Likewise, weak thigh extensors (gluteus maxiumus and hamstring muscles) allow the long leg side innominate bone to subluxate anteriorly, superiorly, and laterally, resulting in anterior pelvic cleavage.

There is an unconscious and sustained (if unsuccessful) effort on the part of the postural control mechanism to reduce pelvic torsion through increased thigh flexor tonus on the short leg side and increased extensor tonus on the long leg side. This attempt to restore postural homeostasis is nonetheless unsuccessful: the thigh muscles are hypertonic/futile. The flexors respond to the mild stretch which is exerted upon them in position 2 (the extensors are unaffected) by increasing their tonicity through the activation of the static stretch reflex, thereby decreasing the compliance of the thigh against the table. This increases the height of the foot as described above, so that "the short leg crosses over and gets longer" in position 2.

In D-, hypertonic/effective thigh extensor contraction subluxates the innominate bone into posterior cleavage on the short leg side, whereas thigh flexor hypertonicity subluxates the innominate bone into a state of anterior cleavage on the long leg side. In position 2, the long leg side thigh flexors increase their state of contraction, again through the action of the static stretch reflex. This increases the height of the foot on the involved side, so that "the long leg gets longer" in position 2.

Youngquist et al hypothesized a similar effect in their discussion of the variability of their data in researching an isolation test. They propose that the DPLC may elicit pain in the subject, causing him to react through "muscle guarding or apprehension to protect the area. Any of these could result in unequal pressure of the legs against the examination table or asymmetric hip pressure as the subject attempts to raise one hip off the table slightly in reaction to pain." Interestingly enough, Youngquist et al invoke this effect to explain possible noise in their data, whereas in the current hypertonic/futile, hypertonic/effective model a similar guarding effect becomes the very substance of the data.

Summary

In the larger scheme of things, a clear and dichotomous distinction may be drawn between the D+ and D- pelvic syndromes [appendix]. Both clinical presentations involve pelvic torsion and chronic postural deviation, and yet arise in fundamentally opposite manners and manifest symmetric but opposite parameters:

• D+ results from primary muscle weakness, in which a weakening of the hip flexors allows a posterior drift of the innominate bone on the short leg side. A weakening of the hip extensors allows an anterior drift of the opposite side innominate. D- results from excessive primary muscle contractures, in which overactive hip extensors pull the innominate bone into a posterior cleavage on the short leg side, and overactive hip flexors pull the innominate into an anterior drift on the long leg side.

• In D+ the hip flexors are hypertonic/futile on the short leg side in an ineffective attempt to restore postural homeostasis. In D- they are hypertonic/effective on the long leg side, cleaving the innominate bone anteriorly.

In D+ the short leg side hip extensors are normal in their tonicity, but overwhelm the abnormally weak hip flexors. In D- they are abnormally active and so pull the short leg side innominate bone into a posterior cleavage.

At present it appears on clinical grounds there is a greater likelihood that in D+ the primary lesion is on the side of the posteriorly cleaved innominate bone. In D- the primary lesion is on the side of the anteriorly cleaved innominate bone.

Epidemiological and management considerations

Clinical presentations involving splinting muscle "spasm" (hypertonicity is generally a more accurate term) may tend to present as D-. The patient comes into the office the day after the football game, or perhaps after a weekend of gardening. There's been a slip'n'fall accident, or maybe there's an acute or chronic lumbar IVD syndrome. On the other hand, cases of chronic postural back pain and asymptomatic patients may tend to present as D+. It is not uncommon for normally D+ patients to present on a given day as D- after a precipitating or aggravating incident, but in these cases the typical short leg side tends to remain unchanged.

In both D- and D+ it is beneficial to augment the effects of spinal and pelvic adjustments with a specific program of soft tissue management, including a stretching regimen and a muscle strengthening program. In D- the emphasis is on stretching hypertonic/effective muscles, whereas in D+ the emphasis is on strengthening hypertonic/futile muscles.

Conclusions

This chapter proposed a biomechanical, kinesiological interpretation of the Derifield pelvic leg check (DPLC). After noting that leg length inequality may be artificially produced in *Position 2* (knees flexed) by having the patient exert mild isometric quadriceps contraction, the author described an orthopedic test which follows from this result. The so-called "paper sign" identified the primary side of involvement in cases of pelvic torsion and bolsters the discrimination of D+ from D-. Ultimately, a clear and dichotomous distinction was drawn between the D+ and D- pelvic syndromes, in which the former results from primary muscle weakness and the latter from primary muscle contracture. The DPLC results stem from a guarding response of the hypertonic/futile thigh flexors in D+, and of the hypertonic/effective thigh flexors in D-.

References

1. Thompson, J.C. Thompson Technique Reference Manual. Thompson Educational Workshops SM and Williams Manufacturing: Elgin IL, 1984; 16
2. Fuhr, A.W., Osterbauer, P.J. Interexaminer reliability of relative leg-length evaluations in the prone, extended position. Chiropractic Technique 1989;1(1):13-17
3. Shambaugh, P., Sclafani, L., Fanselow, D. Reliability of the Derifield-Thompson test for leg length inequality, and use of the test to demonstrate cervical adjusting efficacy. J.M.P.T. 1988;11(5); 396
4. Frogley, H.R. The value and validity of the leg check as used the chiropractic profession. Digest of Chiropractic Economics 1987;29(5):24-25

5. Thompson, J.C. Thompson Technique Reference Manual. Thompson Educational Workshops SM and Williams Manufacturing: Elgin IL, 1984; 27

6. Activator Methods. Seminar Work Book. Activator Methods Chiropractic Technique Seminars: Willmar MN, 1985; 16

7. Lawrence, D.J. Chiropractic concepts of the short leg: a critical review. J.M.P.T. 1985; 8(3); 157

8. Friedman, M. The Methodology of Positive Economics. Essays in Positive Economics

9. Thompson, J.C. Thompson Technique Reference Manual. Thompson Educational Workshops, SM and Williams Manufacturing: Elgin IL, 1984; 10

10. Youngquist, M.W., Fuhr, A.W., Osterbauer, P.J. Interexaminer reliability of an isolation test for the identification of upper cervical subluxation. J.M.P.T. 1989; 12(2);95

11. Magee, D.J. Orthopedic Physical Assessment. W.B. Saunders Company: Phil., 1987; 306

12. Guyton, A.C. Textbook of Medical Physiology. 6th ed. W.B. Saunders: Philadelphia, 1981; 633

13. Christensen, K.D. Clinical Chiropractic Biomechanics. Educational Division Foot Levelers, Inc. Dubuque, 1984; 28, 151

14. Guyton, A.C. Textbook of Medical Physiology. 6th ed. Philadelphia: W.B. Saunders, 1981; 630

15. Walther, D.S. Applied Kinesiology. Volume I. Basic Procedures and Muscle Testing. Systems DC, Pueblo, 1981; 59

16. Hildebrandt, R.W. Chiropractic Spinography. A Manual of Technology and Interpretation. 2nd ed. Williams and Wilkins, Baltimore, 1985; 117

17. Cooperstein, R. Chiropraxis. Self-published, Oakland, 1990; 76.

18. Kendall, F.P., McCreary, E.K. Muscles Testing and Function. 3rd ed. Baltimore/London: Williams & Wilkins, 1983; 270

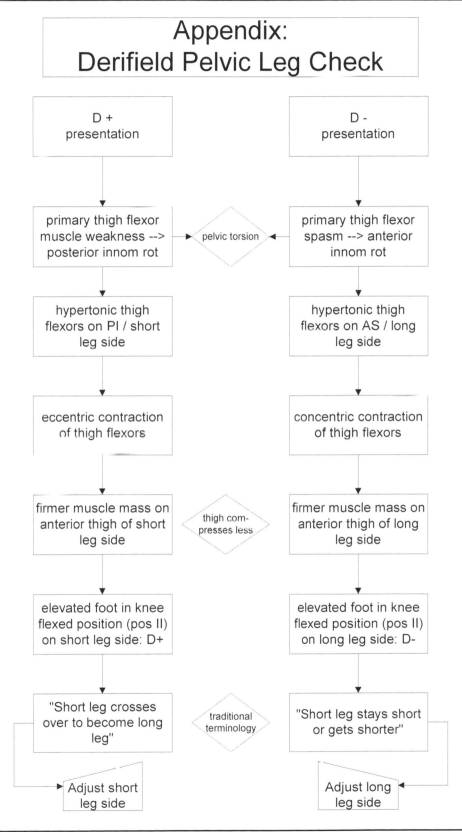

Appendix:
Derifield Pelvic Leg Check

D +
presentation

D -
presentation

primary thigh flexor muscle weakness --> posterior innom rot

pelvic torsion

primary thigh flexor spasm --> anterior innom rot

hypertonic thigh flexors on PI / short leg side

hypertonic thigh flexors on AS / long leg side

eccentric contraction of thigh flexors

concentric contraction of thigh flexors

firmer muscle mass on anterior thigh of short leg side

thigh com-presses less

firmer muscle mass on anterior thigh of long leg side

elevated foot in knee flexed position (pos II) on short leg side: D+

elevated foot in knee flexed position (pos II) on long leg side: D-

"Short leg crosses over to become long leg"

traditional terminology

"Short leg stays short or gets shorter"

Adjust short leg side

Adjust long leg side

11. Adjusting the lumbar spine and pelvis

This chapter will discuss treating lumbopelvic complaints, with and without associated torsion (see the algorithm in the appendix to the chapter). There is an appendix at the end of the chapter summarizing examination findings and appropriate interventions. A rationale and method of adjusting the thoracolumbar region in the supine position is described in the subsequent chapter 'Vectored thoracolumbar adjustments." This chapter emphasizes manipulative procedures, there being separate chapters on blocking and drop table approaches.

Optimization criteria

It must first be pointed out that the lumbar subluxation may be considered segmentally, in the traditional sense, or (especially in the spirit of the preceding chapters) the "subluxation" may be stretched in a sense to refer to the entire lumbopelvic distortion when there is a coherent distortion. In the figure, the subluxation may be understood to include the entire lumbopelvis in distortion. Although not identical to Logan's description, we have at times called this "The Basic Distortion." This would include elements in the sagittal plane, such as alterations in the pelvic carrying angle (PCA), and also in the frontal plane, such as pelvic obliquity and lateral curvatures of the spine. It is best to take these multiplanar effects into account in executing lumbopelvic adjustments, as is made more clear in the text to follow.

It is possible to delimit a slough of "listings" that are inherent to the Basic Distortion. Although any may be performed without harming the patient, provided the identification and its sidedness is correct, it may be the case that some are more worth doing than others. We are presented more or less with a menu of possibilities, with the mandate of choosing those most likely to have the largest beneficial impact upon the patient. Much of the discussion that follows is aimed at deciding how to choose particular interventions as opposed to others. Probably, there is no "best" way. The

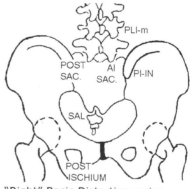

"Right" Basic Distortion, using Logan's phrase (his a little different. Representative listings given.

distortion presents as a postural syndrome, implying that to a large extent we are dealing with a series of coherent findings, rather than one essential cause.

Likewise, there may be multiple paths of approaching and rectifying the syndrome. Each separate component of the lumbopelvic postural complex may retain a holographic trace of the entire entity, which latter may be effectively addressed through any or each separate component. If there is any truth in the oft-heard dictum that "all techniques work," might it not follow from considerations such as these?

Although we will be going through adjustive strategies mostly pertinent to this Basic Distortion, we must keep in mind that there are "segmental patients" as well, those whose low back condition is best understood and addressed from a segmental, specific point of view. The primary segmental contacts used for adjusting the adjusting the lumbosacral area in side-posture (other approaches would have to be mechanically consistent) are represented in the next figure. Although all these moves accomplish a different mechanical result, they remain mechanically consistent with another. They address the same distortion at different points of access. In the discussion that follows, we introduce a number of considerations that bear on choosing adjustive strategies that are optimal. The adjustive procedures themselves come later in the chapter. From time to time, specific adjustive procedures are mentioned, although more formal discussion of the adjustments comes closer to the end of this chapter. Although this discussion occurs in the context of the lumbopelvis, many of the points that are made are equally applicable, in that general points are being made, to the other regions of the spine. For example, the discussion of hypermobility and hypomobility applies to all regions of the spine, and not just the lumbopelvis.

These are some of the factors that are taken into account in account in making selections from the menu of possibilities: postural findings, hypo- and hypermobility, symptomatology, the Derifield result, reflex challenges, and the principles of mechanical advantage. No attempt is herein made to rank the relative importance of these factors. Very often they point coherently toward a specific area to adjust, but at other times they point toward different (but not necessarily inharmonious) areas. In these cases it would be perfectly appropriate to do more than one adjustive procedure, including on a given office visit. The key point to remember is that if the general distortion is correctly pegged, then any of the particular listings that are chosen to be addressed will be "correct" - that is, will not harm the patient, since the LODs will all be directed toward postural neutrality - even though some might be more optimal than others. Particular choices would not so much be wrong as sub-optimal.

I had a little trouble with my side-posture pelvic adjustments, and more than a little trouble with my lumbar segmental adjustments, until I discovered that the key to success involved breaking a few "rules": throwing in a little rotation, a little scissoring, and stabilizing the patient at his crossed arms instead of at the shoulder. There are whole articles out there explaining why it is OK to employ rotational vectors in side-posture adjustments, the critics notwithstanding, the prohibition of which probably devolves from a careless recitation of Harry Farfan's warnings, who seems to have misinterpreted his own work. There may be a need to go into this further, but certainly no time as I hasten to get into the lumbopelvic moves!

Mechanical advantage

If the doctor is small, or the patient is large and/or very fixated, all other things being equal, more leverage will be required. If the doctor is relatively strong and/or large, and the patient small and/or flexible, then less leverage is required. Indeed, in these latter circumstances, larger leverage may not be entirely safe. Of course, this applies not only to the lumbopelvic region but to the cervical and thoracic regions as well. The head and jaw makes a very long lever for some types of cervical adjusting, and the pelvis for some types of low

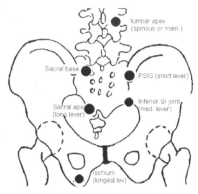

Principal contact points for lumbosacral manipulation, each with varying degrees of mechanical advantage

back adjustments. There is a tradeoff between length of lever and specificity, which may or may not be a problem, depending on what is the nature of the clinical problem and the intent of the procedure. Moreover, long leverage does not always equate to lack of precision: leverage may amplify prestress while the contact hand maintains the specificity that is desired. In the low back area, the sacral apex and iliac blades make for long levers, and the lumbar contacts and sacral base are shorter levers. These are discussed below.

Stabilizing at the patient's crossed arms focuses all the pre-stress over a very narrow number of vertebra, considerably improving upon the more common shoulder stabilization, which dissipates all that great prestress over 24 bones. It is very useful for those hypermobile patients in whom it is difficult to achieve adequate prestress, although I always wonder why we would even want to manipulate these people, since immobilization might be kinder. The thrust is accomplished using both arms and with the doctor's thigh on the patients other thigh. We should avoid conventional unwisdoms like "scissoring bad," "rotation bad." A study should be designed to disprove the null hypothesis, that such procedures are risky, before we toss out such useful parameters in lumbar segmental adjusting.

Rotation: What's the big deal?

One of the most peculiar phenomena I have observed in chiropractic is the exaggerated fear of using rotational pre-stress or line of drive in adjusting the lumbopelvic area. "Rotation" has become a code-word for some sort of deliberately misanthropic and dangerous hatred for patients, as though the doctor using it were actually trying to herniate the disk. One of these days I will have to go through the history of this irrationality, which appears to result from the interplay of several factors:

• a misinterpretation of Farfan's in vitro work demonstration that rotation and compression combined is destructive to the disk;

• the desire to find pseudoscientific justification for what one already does, with pure emotion passing for reason;

• abject fear and loathing of all other adjusting styles other than one's own.

No claim is made that the moves presented in the analysis to follow provide a complete repertoire. They do not. They just happen to be "bread and butter" maneuvers with applicability to most patient presentations. Chiropractic adjustive procedures are usually named and presented according to the name of the maneuver, but I usually (not always) find it more useful to identify the patient contacts to be employed. I am not trying to cover all the styles out there, just the ones I happen to prefer. Sometimes we wind up preferring procedures not so much because we believe them best, but because it just so happens that we were exposed to or mastered them first; the "believing them to be the best moves" part comes later.

Essentially, there are prone, supine, and side-posture approaches to adjusting the lumbar spine, sometimes using adjunctive equipment such as the knee-chest table, padded wedges, and drop-tables. Since I don't return to the knee-chest table anywhere in this text, I should herein comment that the lumbothoracic junctional area is something of a mortise joint, engineered to flex but not extend very much; therefore, the patient's knees should be kept quite cephalad in the knee-chest position, to avoid excessive hyperextension of this area when the thrust is applied. The drop-table moves and blocking with padded wedges procedures get their own chapters below.

The upper lumbars are not quite as amenable to side-posture adjusting as the lower lumbar segments. For this reason, I usually address them using a maneuver that resembles the anterior thoracic adjustment, which becomes in this case an anterior lumbar adjustment. This procedure and the clinical rationale upon which it is based is described in a separate chapter on the lumbothoracic junctional area.

PSIS contact

Since the axis of rotation for the SI joint is near S2, with respect to the SI joint, a PSIS contact employs a very short lever arm, the force being applied very close to the joint. At the same time, with respect to the axis for interinnominate rotation, the symphysis pubis, this contact applies long leverage. This chapter discusses only side posture moves, drop-table and blocking with padded wedges approaches being described in separate chapters.

Modified Pettibon maneuver

I call this a "modified" Pettibon maneuver, because although the basic mechanical style is taken from his work, as exemplified in his proprietary Biomechanics Technique, the LOD and the mechanical intent upon which it is based are, in a word, modified according to my own sense of what needs to be done. Pettibon saw this move has flexing the pelvis on the lumbar spine, whereas my intent is more based on introducing interinnominate rotation. The patient is positioned in side-posture with the posteriorly rotated ilium side up. The spine is placed in a smooth kyphotic arc, with the ipsilateral shoulder pushed somewhat posteriorly and the down-side shoulder pulled somewhat caudally. The doctor may stabilize the patient by pushing up and back at the ipsilateral shoulder, by cupping under and pulling caudally the down-side shoulder, or by pushing against the patient's overlapped hands near his xiphoid area. The doctor draws very near the patient, such that his own sternum is very close and actually touching his contact hand on the patient's PSIS. The "thrust" is accomplished not so much by jabbing the contacting pisiform at the PSIS, but rather through a sudden shifting of the doctor's center of gravity. This is done by swinging the hips cephalad, in a smooth rocking motion. The LOD is P to A, I to 5, and somewhat M to L by virtue of the fact that the patient is very much rolled underneath the doctor's contact hand. It must be emphasized that this contact hand does not so much deliver the thrust as aim and focus it. The thrust actually comes from the entire body, especially the swing of the hips. This is not the best move when there is a clinical presumption of disc herniation, because it has a flexion quality, at least in the prestress.

Diversified side-posture, or body drop maneuver

To call this a "Diversified side posture" move is less a question of what it is, and more a question of what it is not: it is not a Gonstead-like procedure which eschews rotation, is very arm oriented, stabilizes at the patient's upside shoulder; and introduces primarily extension forces. On the contrary, the patient is pre-positioned with some degree of lumbopelvic rotation; the doctor stabilizes on the patient's crossed forearms, where a watch may be worn; the thrust is accomplished by the doctor dropping onto the patient's thigh, aiming somewhat caudally so as not to simply compress the pelvis on the table, with his or her own thigh; and the thrust may add rotation to the extension vector. The rotation should be well tolerated, in the prestress and in the thrust, at least if the Basic Distortion is present,

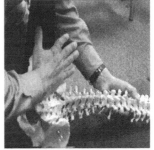

Sacral notch contact.

because this move unwinds the helical component of the distortion. I once wrote an article (see next chapter) entitled "Would you believe a $50.00 roll?" more or less about this move, in which I made the point that this move descends from the infamous "million dollar roll," but differs from it in that there is a specific contact, it matters which side is up (the side of posterior innominate rotation), and the amount of rotation introduced is judiciously selected – that is, is not excessive. The thigh on thigh or "pocket-to-pocket" element of this setup is understood just as it is in the Gonstead technique, although unlike in Gonstead, this element of the adjustive procedure is not confined to the AS ilium situation.

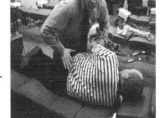

Body-drop, PSIS contact.

In the end, three forces are introduced at the moment of truth: a thrust back on the patient's crossed forearms, a vigorous drop on the patient's thigh, and a thrust on the PSIS. This PSIS thrust, rather than being the prime mover as in some side posture styles, more or less establishes a fixed point between the thrust on the forearms and the drop on the patient's thigh. If the pre-positioning is uncomfortable for the patient, either the wrong side is up, the doctor having got the helical component of the distortion wrong (confounded anterior for posterior torsion of the involved side). Or, perhaps the doctor is doing what he or she wants to do, and the listing is correct, but the patient simply can't tolerate the torsion in the rib cage for whatever reason.

Sacral notch contact

Either the modified Pettibon or Diversified side-posture approach works well. Relative to the SI joint, this moves applies more leverage than the PSIS contact, because the force is applied some 1.5 inches from the probable joint axis. Again, the posteriorly rotated ilium side is up. The set-up and "thrust" are more or less the same as in the PSIS contact (therefore no need for an illustration of the thrust procedure), except that the LOD is more inferior to superior. The pisiform of the doctor's contact hand is positioned in the soft tissue just inferior to the sacroiliac joint, in the cleft between the innominate bone and the sacral border. In a certain sense the sacroiliac joint has "gone inferior," and this move simply hoists it up. Because the contact is further from any manipulable joints, the cavitation events that occur are less precisely identifiable. This may or may not be a problem, depending on the goals of the practitioner. When the patient needs to be flexed, or at least adjusted in flexion, this move is more on that path than the otherwise similar move described above using a PSIS contact.

Sacral apex contact

I have not found the Diversified side-posture setup to work very well for this move, so I tend to use the modified Pettibon maneuver. Among side-posture low back moves, this one has the longest lever. The indications for the move include not only pelvic torsion, but the need to hyperflex the patient, since a contact so low in the pelvis cannot fail to introduce flexion. The intent is to straighten out a deviated sacral apex, which automatically elevates the contralateral sacral base, which has subluxated inferiorly. This move is actually a side-posture equivalent to Thompson's SAL and SAR maneuvers, which he performs in the prone position and on a drop-table. It descends to some extent from Pettibon's "#2" set-up. It is an especially opportune maneuver when the patient exhibits lumbosacral hyperextension. If there is pelvic torsion, it is applied to the side of anterior innominate rotation, since it has the character of an

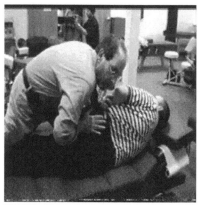
Modified Pettibon deimbrication move, sacral apical area.

AS ilium move, since the thrust is applied low in the pelvis. If there is no appreciable pelvic torsion, the move may be applied to either side. The set-up is similar to that described for the PSIS and sacral notch. The "thrust," again, is actually a swing of the hips with the doctor's sternal area in close contact with the his contact hand, which more or less envelops the entire sacrum, but favors the upside lateral border. The LOD is primarily lateral to medial, with a P to A component as well.

A slight variation in the set-up for the sacral apex move optimizes it for the treatment of stable spondylolisthetic spondylolisthesis. The contact hand would be centered perpendicular to the sacral apex, rather than arranged along the sacral border. The LOD is more straight P to A than lateral to medial. Pettibon offers a rationale for the value of this maneuver that has ultimately to do with traction on the PLL, which allegedly straightens out interruptions in George's line.

The sacral apex move may also be used to treat an anterior subluxation of the coccyx, following a hard landing on the buttocks. In this variation on the same theme, the thrust is directed just superior to the sacrococcygeal joint, in an effort to extend the joint. The patient is asked to hold his or her breath on full inspiration, to maintain some degree of centripetal force, to provide resistance for the centrifugal force generated by the doctor's thrust. (Take into account that the patient is likely to pass some wind.) If the coccyx is subluxated laterally as well, the patient would be adjusted with side of the sacrococcygeal joint open wedge up, in side posture.

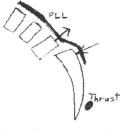

Thrusting near sacral apex tensions the PLL, tending to realign the lumbosacral spine

Another means of correcting an anterior coccyx involves a sustained tugging force from inferior to superior on the prone patient' coccyx, using the thumb of the superior hand to get a grip and pull, and the heel of the other hand to apply a strong push to the thumb. This procedure would be known as the "Diversified Coccyx" adjustment.

Sacral base

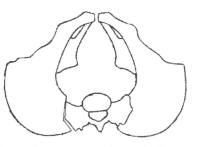

Diversified coccyx adjustment, Peterson

The sacral base can subluxate "on its own" in relation to both innominate bones, a primary sacral subluxation; or it can subluxate as part of the pelvic torsion syndrome, as a compensation. In the case of compensatory sacral sublxuation, although one could adjust the sacrum, it usually suffices to simply take care of the torsion and let the sacrum then take care of itself. In the case of primary sacral subluxation, the sacral base may subluxate either anterior or posterior in relation to an innominate bone. One would suppose that usually the sacrum subluxates anteriorly, either unilaterally or bilaterally, owing to the fact that there is less resistance to it dropping into the pelvic bowl than there is in it moving posteriorly. It is not obvious how an anterior-inferior sacrum could be addressed through a contact on the sacral base, but this author is not unaware of such efforts. A P to A contact on the sacral base when it

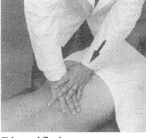

Posterior sacrum on innominate wedges ilia apart, probably not most common SI subluxation.

subluxates posteriorly, on the other hand, is a rather obvious strategy.

The sacrum, when it subluxates posteriorly, brutally forces the innominate bones apart by a powerful wedge action, since it is wider at its anterior aspect. The so-called "posterior-inferior sacrum" (I am not sure it is inferior at all) occurs on the long leg side, as the sacrum counternutates there in response to innominate AS rotation. These subluxations are quite painful, due to the fact that the sacrum wedges the ilia apart when it migrates posteriorly. The stretch in the posterior sacroiliac ligament is presumably the pain generator. When a patient comes in with a bona fide posterior-sacrum (aka posterior sacral base), he or she is hurting! Let us recall Diane Lee's comment that counternutation breeds instability, and no doubt allows this subluxation to occur These are my low back "throwing-away-the-crutch" patients, some of best chiromiracles.

The patient is set up in side-posture, usually with the involved sacroiliac joint side down (for the purpose of stabilizing it with the patient's own body weight). Then a thrust is delivered at the sacral base, and that's that . . . usually. If it doesn't work, the doctor can try thrusting with the involved side up. And if that doesn't work, a prone drop-table move would be the next thing to try.

An appendix at the end of this chapter addresses primary and compensatory sacral subluxation, both the palpatory examination procedure and suggested clinical interventions.

Lumbar spinal contacts

My preferred lumbar move is more or less identical to the body drop (Diversified side-posture) as described above for the PSIS contact, except the contact this time is on a lumbar vertebra. It is best applied to L3-5, although it can be performed with less precision on L1-2, bones I prefer to adjust using the vectored lumbar anterior maneuver described in a later chapter. Although much is commonly made of how the hand is held – fingers up the spine for "rotatory" scoliosis, or across the spine for "simple" scoliosis – the simple truth is that using this style, the adjusting hand is very weak if the fingers do not cross the spine.

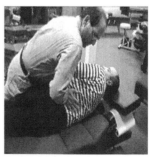

Body drop, lumbar segmental.

The modified Pettibon maneuver can be performed in the lower lumbars, but being aware of a case in which a patient's shoulder was separate, I no longer consider that an ideal choice of moves. One would never wish to overgeneralize from one negative experience, but the move seems rather difficult to control with a sternal drop so far from the doctor's center of gravity. This is a point made only withy great difficulty in prose, but which is utterly obvious in a laboratory situation. As has already been stated, it is prudent to switch over to a more P to A, classic Gonstead-like setup (the reader may consult Dr. Plaugher's book[1] favoring extension, when the patient appears to have a herniated disc. I do not take the trouble to describe this setup, since it is so well-known and is well-described in virtually any textbook of chiropractic.

The big ugly

This paragraph, unlike the others, is oriented toward a maneuver, rather than taking as its theme a particular contact. There are times when, all the doctor's good intentions notwithstanding, nothing seems to work, or the doctor simply anticipates that the cards are stacked against him even prior to attempting the side-posture move. Enter *The Big Ugly*, so-named by a teaching associate who once heard me paraphrasing Pettibon: "when you are mud wrestling with ole man sub, nothing is too ugly!" In the Big Ugly, the doctor places one knee on the table, behind the patient's buttocks. The doctor's superior arm controls the patient's downside shoulder, with forearm across the patient's chest, and inferior pisiform is applied to the patient's PSIS or sacral apical area. From there, the doctor does whatever it takes to aim his or her torso into the contact hand, as described above as the modified Pettibon move. All bets are off as to the exact LOD, or juxtaposition of patient and doctor body parts: this move will take whatever it takes. This move should not be applied to any level above the sacral base, if that; things start to unravel quickly in terms of what mechanics are introduced by the move.

---

[1] Plaugher G, editor. Textbook of clinical chiropractic: a specific biomechanical approach. Baltimore, Maryland: Williams & Wilkins; 1993.

Appendix: Lumbopelvic protocol

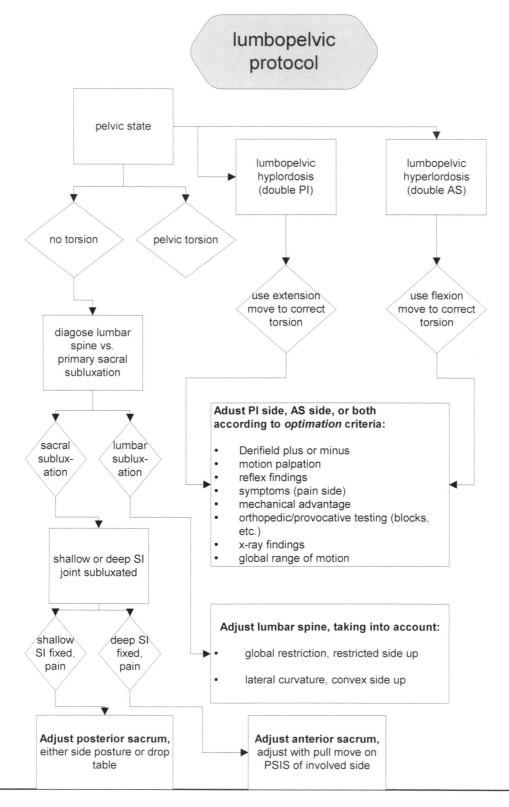

Appendix: Interpretation of sacral base palpatory findings

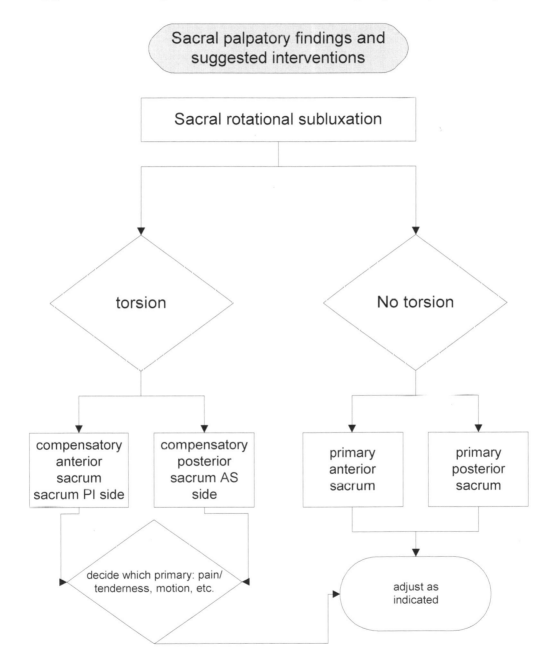

12. Would you believe a *Fifty Dollar* roll?[1]

In a profession rarely bereft of spectacle, one of the most awesome sights remains chiropractors adjusting one another on the exhibiting floor of a state convention. The table vendors like to have their consultants adjusting anything that moves, hoping to attract an enthusiastic crowd of adjustees and spectators that will draw attention to the tables.

Obviously, there are a lot of things wrong with this. What makes for good business does not necessarily make for good chiropractic. These consultants, who like most other chiropractors would like themselves seen as portal of entry and even primary care providers, do not pay much attention to details—you know, little things, like taking a history, performing an examination, and ruling out contraindications prior to adjusting the spine. At state conventions, all that doctor stuff plays second fiddle to the solitary goal of producing audibles loud enough to hypnotize an adoring crowd amidst the din and cacophony of the exhibitor area.

A chiropractic student, having observed this same phenomenon at technique seminars, launches a remark into cyberspace: "It is amazing to me that when chiropractors go to a seminar and ask one another to give them an adjustment, it only takes a minute or two, but if you do this with a patient then you are considered irresponsible. Where is the logic here?" Dr. Badanes answers: "Apparently, no one (really) takes VS and Subluxation less seriously than chiropractors themselves . . . When you treat a person, whether they are a chiropractor, baker, Indian chief, or your mother, at a party, seminar, or in a restaurant bathroom, it is bad practice to assume anything other than that they are your patient at those times."

But let us not dwell upon the undoctorly conduct of these convention doctors, for that is not my main point. Rather, let us fast forward to a matter of *pure technique,* the style these doctors tend to use. Neither of the two chiropractic colleges where I have taught allowed low back moves such as these: the patient's upper leg is draped over the edge of the table and used as a crank to turn the low back, while the doctor simultaneously propels the shoulder up and away, or even pins it square to the table. There may not even be a contact hand somewhere on the low back or sacroiliac area.

---

[1] This chapter is based on an article that was originally published in *Dynamic Chiropractic.*

This rather dramatic counter-rotation of the shoulder and pelvic girdles, the so called "million dollar roll" (so-named because doctors who employ it become millionaires?), although generally relegated to the dinosaur department in technique classes, public discussion, and probably most technique seminars, is clearly alive and well on the convention floor. Judging from the appreciative swooning of the observers, and the dazed expression of gratitude that generally adorns the subject's face as he staggers away from the table ("Thanks doc, I really needed that. . .") I would suspect that the million dollar roll is also alive and well in many chiropractic offices around the country.

"The most dangerous technique in spinal manipulation is excessive rotation of the spinal column," so writes a famous doctor. Perhaps, but even when a given procedure is "the most dangerous" relative to others, it does not follow that it is dangerous in the absolute, any more than saying "the most common color of Edsels is white" means there must be lots of white Edsels rolling around. Although I must remain agnostic on the relative danger of rotational lumbar moves, never having seen any data one way or the other, I would be very surprised were they to be found dangerous. If indeed they were, the daily carnage in chiropractic offices around the country would have surfaced by now, and possibly even put an end to the profession.

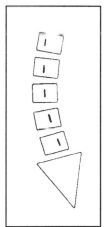

Helical nature of lumbar lateral curvature, left PI configuration.

There is good reason to believe that a rotational vector in lumbar side posture adjustments may not only be safe, but *indicated* insofar as it addresses the helical component of the overall lumbopelvic distortion. Hugh Logan's observation (1), that when the sacral base subluxates inferiorly, the lumbar spine assumes a lateral curvature convex on the ipsilateral side, has been confirmed many times. Johnston (2) pointed out from a theoretical point of view that the lumbar adaptation would take the form of a spiral, while Friberg (3) confirmed this helical nature of the lumbar lateral curvature through quantitative radiographic analysis. In the figure, although the lower lumbar spinous processes are to the left of the central ray of the x-ray, each spinous process is to the right of the spinous process of the segment below.

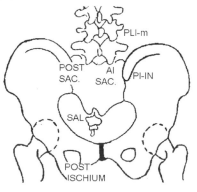

The inferiority of the sacrum is not a stand-alone finding. The entire suite of positional derangements is seen in the figure, which illustrates an AI sacrum right, SAL, PI-

IN ilium right, AS-EX ilium left, and multiple lumbar segmental misalignments of the PLI-m persuasion. Although a strict chiropractic segmentalist would have to find a way to decide which of these listings is primary, a chiropractic structuralist (4) might see the entire set of osseous positional derangements as the subluxation: a left lumbopelvic basic distortion, in Logan's sense. The structuralist could also detect yet another listing: a multisegmental Y axis helical distortion. If we regard the adjustment is segmentally specific, then by comparison the helical component of the distortion is addressed by a *vectored manipulation*.

Patients, while neither theoreticians nor radiometrically inclined, are intuitively aware of this helical twist in their subluxated lumbopelvic spines, at least judging from their propensity to self-manipulate it. Once in a while, a patient will ask me if it is OK to twist their own backs and make popping noises. Before I furiously denounce her for being reckless with her own spine, or even for practicing chiropractic without a license, I do at least ask to be shown how she does it. Sitting on my table, she may lean backwards and drag her left knee across the night, keeping her left shoulder planted near the table; or maybe she stands up with her hands clasped near the sternum, and suddenly swings her elbows to the left while jerking her flexed left knee up and away to the right. If my descriptions are hard to visualize, just think of Chubby

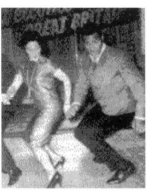

Chubby Checker and friend self-manipulating using bilateral, weight-bearing lumbar roll procedure.

Checker (or anyone else) doing the twist, either supine or in the weight-bearing position. By his own description, the dance requires that you "put out a cigarette with both feet and wipe your bottom with a towel."

Although Chubby Checker remains a bilateral twister, the typical patient will tell you that she generally performs her self-manipulation maneuver in one direction only, or at least only one direction produces pops and affords relief. Which direction? Turning toward the side of her left PI-IN ilium, of course. In the standing position, friction of her feet with the floor keeps the pelvic girdle relatively stationery, while she rotates her shoulder girdle posteriorly on the left. Swinging her flexed left knee to the right would accentuate the effect.

The chiropractor, adjusting her left PI-IN ilium, would exert some degree of posterior pressure on the left shoulder, while thrusting the pelvic girdle anteriorly on the left. A moment's reflection will confirm that the patient and the chiropractor achieve the same relative opposed rotation of the shoulder and pelvic girdles. The doctor emphasizes an anterior thrust on the left pelvic girdle, while the patient emphasizes a posterior tug on the left shoulder girdle. I point this out not to encourage self-manipulation, but only to draw out the mechanical, diagnostic significance of the vectors that patients use in their instinctive attempt to unwind the *helical component of their lumbopelvic postural distortion.*

In my practice, I have developed this observation into an orthopedic sign. The standing patient is asked to clasp his hands at the waist and then rotate his torso to the end point of motion, first to the left and then to the right. One direction (toward the PI side) will subjectively feel more comfortable to the patient or exhibit less strain at the end point than the other. He will explain that rotation to the less favored side puts greater strain on the foot, knee, low back, and ribcage, or just feels "yucky."

The famous doctor continues: "We wouldn't want to be associated with a doctor who lumbar-rolls a patient both sides." Although excommunication seems too harsh a sentence for the aficionado of the bilateral lumbar roll, given the lack of outcomes-based evidence on the matter, it remains likely that one direction of thrust unwinds the helical component of the patient's lumbar distortion, whereas the other

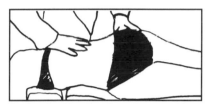

Farfan testing torsion. Aggravation of pain would bar left PI ilium move (from Markey).

direction aggravates it. I continue to be amazed by how shortsightedly some chiropractors would make pariahs out of brethren whose moves they happen to dislike, even though they have stood the test of time (e.g., rotatory cervical moves and lumbar rolls), thus providing ammunition to outside detractors. (Once I found a new patient recruitment leaflet in the meat section of a local supermarket, produced by a fellow chiropractor whom I knew well, explaining how she uses safe and effective treatment methods, unlike those other chiropractors who adjust the spine using "violent, sudden, dangerous twists and jerks." Nice.)

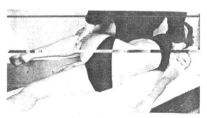

Cyriax manipulating for lumbar disc lesion.

Although I am obviously making a case for a limited version of the lumbar roll, it would seem prudent, *ceteris paribus*, to stick to one side for most patients. Medical manipulator Harry Farfan tested lumbopelvic torsion bilaterally prior to manipulating, counter-rotating the shoulder girdle and pelvic girdle of the prone patient in an opposed manner as an orthopedic test, thus determining the preferred line of drive. Chiropractors generally perform this type of test with the patient in side posture: we simply call it *setting up on the patient*, or testing the adjustment prior to thrusting.

Another medical manipulator, James Cyriax, advocated highly rotated lumbar manipulation ("Applying a rotation strain is a very effective way of securing reduction at a low lumbar level.") as a treatment for lumbar disc herniation, and often performed it with the patient under anesthesia – sometimes using an assistant to increase the leverage. He believed that twisting or flexion of the spine would tighten up the posterior longitudinal ligament, so that its tension would exert a posteroanterior (centripetal) force upon the bulging annular fibers and nucleus pulposus. Chiropractor James Cox has also invoked spinal flexion as a parallel strategy to tighten up the posterior longitudinal ligament, and for the same purpose (5).

How dangerous is this rotation? Farfan (6), who found that he could herniate a cadaveric lumbar disc using a combination of compression and rotation, is often invoked to support this prohibition of rotation. Nevertheless, he found that the facets would have to fracture before he could produce enough intersegmental rotation to herniate a disc, both in normal and degenerated spines. Furthermore, the pattern of disc herniation he achieved (laminar separation) did not resemble the typical radial fissures seen in real patients. Whatever clinical conclusions Farfan drew from his own work as to manipulative strategies, Cassidy et al (7) use these same data to defend the safety of sensible rotational vectors in side-posture lumbar manipulation.

One of the most peculiar phenomena I have observed in chiropractic is contempt for the practice of using rotational pre-stress or lines of drive in adjusting the spine, including the lumbopelvic area. *Rotation* in some quarters has become a code-word for some sort of deliberately misanthropic and dangerous hatred for patients, as though the doctor using it were actually trying to herniate the disc. Sure, a "million dollar roll" does seem a bit much . . . but would you believe a *fifty dollar roll,* on one side only, maybe using a contact hand?

Notes

1. Logan HB. Textbook of Logan Basic Methods. St. Louis, Missouri: 1950. (Logan VF, Murray FM, eds.
2. Johnston LC. The paradox of the functional spine. Journal of the Canadian Chiropractic Association 1966(June-July):7-10.
3. Friberg O. Leg length inequality and low back pain. Clinical Biomechanics 1987;2:211-219.
4. Rosenthal MJ. The structural approach to chiropractic: from Willard Carver to present practice. Chiropractic History 1981;1(1):25-29.

5. Cox JM. Low back pain, mechanism, diagnosis and treatment. (4th ed.) Baltimore MD: Williams & Wilkins, 1985.

6. Farfan HF. Mechanical disorders of the low back. Philadelphia: Lea & Febiger, 1973.

7. Cassidy JD, Thiel HW, Kirkaldy-Willis WH. Side posture manipulation for lumbar intervertebral disk herniation. Journal of Manipulative and Physiological Therapeutics 1993;16:96-103.

13. Drop-table lumbopelvic procedures

In a preceding chapter we discussed side-posture manipulative procedures for the lumbopelvis. In this chapter, we discuss drop-table adjusting, and in the next, the use of padded wedges. Ideally speaking, we would have data as to which particular adjustive procedures get the best outcome, for specific clinical conditions, for given

Indications for drop-table assisted adjusing	
•	Patient too large for side-posture HVLA
•	Side-posture ineffective
•	Avoid rotation (if necessary)
•	Very useful for abnormal sagittal plane curves (double AS/PI)
•	Relative contraindications
•	abdominal aneurysm
•	atherosclerosis

patients, at various moments in the course of their case. Unfortunately, this information is not forthcoming at the present time, and so common sense will have to do, based upon our clinical experience and the small amount of evidence we do have. I will have to turn to these matters some other time, because there is no time to linger in this speculative realm just now. An appendix at the end of the chapter illustrates the implementation of drop table examination and treatment procedures as performed in the Pierce-Stillwagon Technique.

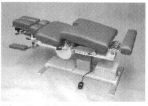

The Zenith Hi-Lo table. Can be elevated.

Historical considerations

Although the Thompson Technique does not equal drop-table technique, the historical situation should be acknowledged. At the current time, drop-tables are so taken for granted that it is difficult to realize how central the invention of the Terminal Point table was to the development of the Thompson technique. According to Moulton, J. Clay Thompson headed research and development at the Palmer College for over 10 years, working closely with B.J. Palmer in the development of the first drop headpiece in 1952. Dr. Quigley brought the headpiece to his Clearview Sanitorium, where he used it with great results on his mental patients. Thompson constructed the first table incorporating cervical, dorsolumbar, and pelvic drop pieces in 1957.

Thompson states: "By eliminating spinal subluxations in an organized, orderly fashion, from 'top down and inside out,' the Thompson practitioner will begin to verify the corrections he is making on the patient's spine." At the heart of the technique is the Derifield leg check, adapted from the original work of Dr. Romer Derifield from Detroit, Michigan. The leg check procedure purports to detect neurophysiological imbalance, resulting from subluxations, as manifested by a "contractured leg." The Thompson "Terminal Point" table aims not only at protecting the patient from being over-adjusted, but at promoting the clinical longevity of the doctor.

If the drop-table is central to Thompson's technological innovations, then his leg check procedure is analogously central to his analytic contributions. He adapted it from the work of Dr. Romer Derifield, who discovered quite fortuitously that prone leg lengths occasionally changed when the patient rotated his head. Further investigation by Derifield revealed that thrusting into tender nodules in the (mostly upper) cervical spine would not only reduce the patient's symptomatology but ameliorate prone LLI.

Pierce-Stillwagon Technique (PST)[1] follows in the tradition of Thompson technique, and therefore retains much of it flavor: the importance of a Derifield-derived leg check procedure, the emphasis on the cervical and pelvic areas, and heavy reliance on drop tables. To the Thompson analysis are added two important pelvic listings (Double PI and Double AS) and one important cervical listing (Fifth Cervical). There is much greater emphasis on the role of x-ray and thermography, both as part of the examination procedure and as part of outcome assessment. There is considerable scope for the incorporation of other chiropractic techniques into the scope of PST, including Logan Basic, upper cervical technique, and Reaver's Fifth Cervical technique[2].

In the chapter above on the Derifield leg check, we discussed some of the basic scientific considerations that bear on both the cervical and pelvic syndromes. The cervical syndromes cannot, at least at the present time, be clearly distinguished from the physiology of the normal tonic neck reflex, and will not be further discussed. Pierce's C5 move for lordosis restoration is discussed in the chapter on the neck. I will confine myself herein to the lumbopelvic syndromes.

Biomechanical considerations

---

[1] Pierce WV, Stillwagon G. Pierce-Stillwagon Seminar Manual. Monongahela, Pennsylvania; 1976.

[2] Reaver C. The Fifth Cervical Key. Dravosburg, Pennsylvania: Chirp, Inc.; 1977.

There have been a few articles written the physics of drop-table adjusting, but in the end, little is known about how drop-tables effect patients differently from non-assisted thrust techniques. Most doctors seem to think these moves are safer than side-posture thrust techniques, probably because the magnitude by which the movable piece can drop to some extent limits the distance through which the segmental contact point can be moved. Compare, for example, the amount of extension that can be introduced to the lumbar spine by a knee-chest table or very P to A side-posture maneuver, with what can be introduced by a prone drop-table move.

Whatever difference it makes from a patient point of view, the drop-table makes an indisputable difference from the doctor's point of view: it is easier on the doctor's body. Certainly, the doctor's ability to help patients very much depends on maintaining the ability of the doctor to deliver adjustive thrusts. Drop-table moves are widely considered to conserve the doctor's musculoskeletal integrity, if not the patient's!

One more point needs to be made. A study was done that measured various of the parameters involved in drop-table assisted manipulation. In 1990, Hessel et al[3] measured the forces produced by 2 chiropractors on each of 6 patients, using a drop-table assisted HVLA thrust *intended* to impact upon the PSIS. To put the matter simply, they attempted to correct something that sounds like a PI ilium, using an adjustive procedure attributed to the Thompson Technique. Each subject received 3 thrusts from each chiropractor, 6 in all, with 2 minutes between thrusts and 20 minutes between chiropractors.

The investigators measured 5 parameters: preloading force, peak force, duration of manipulation, impulse of manipulation, and point of application of the peak force. Although all the data were interesting, and mostly consistent with the results of previous studies, I would like to draw attention to just one of the experimental findings: "The location of the point of application of the peak force relative to a low back reference system appeared to be very consistent. However, it was not on the posterior superior iliac spines (PSIS) as expected, but always slightly medial to this point."

Let's see: The peak force was *always* (my emphasis) produced "slightly" medial to the PSIS. Slightly? In fact, as can be seen in the figure, the doctors missed the

---

[3]Hessel BW, Herzog W, Conway PJW, al e. Experimental measurement of the force exerted during spinal manipulation using the Thompson technique. Journal of Manipulative and Physiological Therapeutics 1990;13(8):448-453.

PSIS by 1 to 6 cm, by an average of about 3 cm, landing all over the sacral base!

By any theory of the PI ilium, surely it must be a matter of some consequence to consistently slip medially off the contacted PSIS and wind up thrusting on the sacrum. As it turned out, neither of the two doctors in the study, in attempting to thrust on the PSIS of a prone patient, managed to land even one thrust upon it. They invariably missed, landing on the sacral base. This is a sobering thought. Just when we thought we had a problem with diagnostic specificity, we now learn we may have a companion problem with therapeutic specificity. I can only conclude from this that nothing should be taken for granted, in drop-table or any other type of thrusting technique: in the delivery of the force, it may be very easy to simply slip off the contact and wind up on another segmental contact point altogether. Therefore, we had best be careful to not do so, and find out through more studies if more care lends itself to more precision. I assume nothing. I deal with these matters more thoroughly in an article in Dynamic Chiropractic[4]

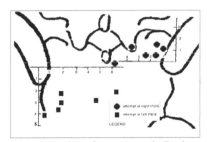

Based on data from Hessel. Each of 12 attempts to adjust the PSIS impacted on the sacrum instead.

Selected drop-table moves

I will not attempt to further distinguish what is Thompson, what is Pierce-Stillwagon, what is whatever else. The honest truth is that the procedures are quite straightforward, and for that reason I will do little more that list out the main procedures and show a few selected illustrations. Some standard drop table moves are not illustrated, but the reader may consult the books by Dr. Zemelka[5] and Dr. Hyman[6] for them, or the Thompson and PST technique manuals cited above. Although not shown in any of the illustrations, nor discussed below, it is helpful to use padded wedges for added mechanical advantage in many (but not all) of the moves described below.

D+ and D-

We discussed D- and D+ situations in the chapter above on the Derifield leg check, and came to the conclusion that the designation ultimately seemed to designate the side of the body that needed to be the focus of attention. Orthodox

---

[4]Cooperstein R. Specificity failure and petrified thought. Dynamic Chiropractic 1999;17(13):20-21, 50-51.

[5] Zemelka WH. The Thompson Technique. Bettendorf, Iowa: Victoria Press; 1992.

[6] Hyman RC. The Thompson Chiropractic Technique: Publisher unknown; 1991.

drop-table practitioners are unlikely to come to that same conclusion, but their clinical practice might not come out that different from what is herein espoused.

For them, the Derifield negative and Derifield positive designations involve posterior-inferior subluxation of the innominate bone, but of somewhat different nature: D+ supposedly involves a translatory subluxation of the innominate bone (one we have previously argued is unlikely) and D- a rotational subluxation of the innominate bone, around the hip (an axis for interinnominate rotation we have judged unlikely).

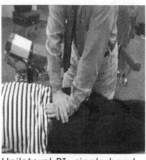

Unilateral PI, single hand contact.

Despite the differences between my interpretation and more conventional interpretations of the Derifield phenomenon, the D+ finding clinically leads to a P to A thrust on the innominate bone, on a drop-table for the practitioners under discussion. For them, the correction of D- requires a two step process, with the first move consisting of a thrust on the ischium of the involved side, and the second move consisting of a thrust upon the inguinal ligament area. Since I have never understood the logic of this correction, and have not used it enough to judge on its clinical effect, it is not part of my repertoire, and I simply remain agnostic on its use. I address D- as described in the chapter on the Derifield leg check, by intervening on the long leg side: an AS ilium, lumbosacral or other lumbar facet problem, etc.

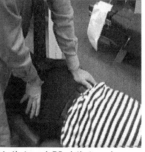

Unilateral PI, bilateral contact.

The upper figure shows a thrust on the PSIS using a single hand contact for correct D+. The lower figure shows a D+ correction, in which the doctor contacts both the PSIS of the involved side and the ischium on the other side. The thrust may be administered a number of times, approximately 3 being typical. The patient's involved side leg may be crossed over the other leg, possibly to relax the involved side piriformis muscle.

There is also a supine PI ilium move (not shown), involving a contact on the involved side pubic bone. I guess I wouldn't mind how invasive this move is for the typical patient if the move were to make mechanical sense. Indeed, if the innominate bone rotated around the hip or SI joint into lesion, as drop-table practitioners seem to believe, this move *would* make sense, because the pubic ramus would subluxate anteriorly as the PSIS subluxated posteriorly. But I don't think this happens, at least not commonly. My "typical" D- correction, as stated previously, may involve a number of possibilities, so no figure is included, other than the AS corrections.

SAL, SAR

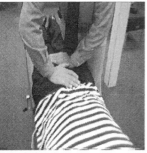

SAL adjustment

SAL and SAR refer to sacral apex left, and sacral apex right, respectively. We have already commented that these listings typically occur as part of the pelvic torsion syndrome, since sacral inferiority, usually associated with torsion, is what automatically creates the deviation of the sacral apex. The figure illustrates the Thompson sacral adjustment. The contact hand is on the sacral apex, adjusting it from lateral to medial. The other hand stabilizes on the sacral base of the short leg side. Personally, since my mechanical analysis indicates that the sacral apex is expected to deviate precisely when there is pelvic torsion, I stabilize on the PSIS, rather than medial to it on the sacral base. I'm not sure that Dr. Thompson would approve. If I really want to take care of sacral apex deviation, I take a straight-away stance and thrust directly lateral to medial on the sacral apex, using the knife edge of my contact point. Clearly, that is the longest possible available lever on the sacrum.

AS ilium

The setup for adjusting the unilateral AS ilium (or posterior ischium, as some would say) is seen in the left and right figures, prone and supine versions respectively. These moves, apart from whatever impact they have on the sacroiliac joints, are likely to deimbricate the lumbar spine; that is, reduce extension there. I prefer the supine version of this move, in which the contact would be applied to the ASIS. Not all patients can tolerate having their ASIS touched, in which case the doctor asks the patient to place a hand on their own ASIS. Then, the doctor's thrust can be applied

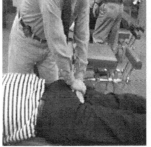

Unilateral AS, prone. Note S to I LOD.

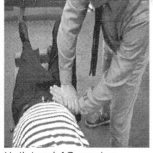

Unilateral AS, supine

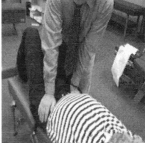

Bilateral AS, supine.

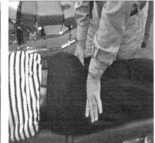

Bilateral AS, prone.

through the patient's own hand. The supine drop-table AS adjustment is the longest possible lever for introducing anterior innominate rotation around the symphysis pubis, for which reason I rarely perform a side-posture AS ilium adjustment.

Double AS, Double PI

In PST technique, there are moves presented for treating bilateral AS and PI iliums. These bilateral listings are not to be interpreted as bilateral sacroiliac lesions, but rather as postural distortions that involve both the pelvis and the lumbar spine. That is, the bilateral AS configuration is associated with lumbar hyperlordosis, and the bilateral PI ilium syndrome is associated with lumbar hypolordosis. The figures show supine (left) and prone (right) setups for the bilateral AS, and a prone bilateral PI adjustment (below). I do not perform or illustrate a supine bilateral

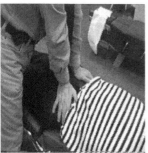

Double PI prone.

PI adjustment, since I can think of better ways to reduce the lumbopelvic lordosis.

Again, the bilateral AS or PI is not primarily a bilateral subluxation of the sacroiliac joint, and therefore the nomenclature is unfortunate, a misnomer because it suggests sacroiliac subluxation. It is diagnosed by the simple x-ray appearance of an anteriorly or posteriorly tipped pelvis (short or long obturator foramina, round or angular pelvic bowl, respectively).

The most effective approach for the bilateral AS is to use a supine set-up, with the pelvic piece set to drop. The patient's knees are flexed. The doctor generally thrusts on the ASISs, using an A to P and I to S LOD, perhaps 3 times. What happens in this adjustment is that the hollow of the lumbar lordosis is flattened on the table, and the pelvis is forced into a posterior rotation. This is a good "deimbrication" protocol, insofar as everything is flexed. Thompson shows this same set-up as an approach to spondylolisthesis, with the doctor's contact on the anterior aspect of the lumbar spine, through the soft tissue of the abdomen. The drop-piece has to be set with light tension for this maneuver. The mechanical advantage for this particular set-up may be improved if a block, or perhaps an SOT-style padded board, is pre-positioned under the

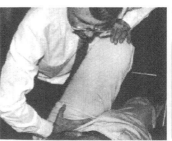

Traditional IN drop table adjustment

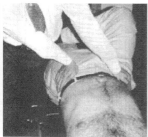

Traditional EX drop table adjustment

patient's pelvis. I prefer the prone to the supine bilateral PI ilium setup, because it appears to achieve a greater reduction in the lumbopelvic lordosis.

IN, EX ilium

There are supine drop moves described for an IN and for an EX ilium. Traditionally, these are performed supine, using the femur of the patient's flexed leg to introduce the forces. Since I am skeptical of the analysis that goes into the listings, I do not perform these moves; I believe IN ilums go along with the territory of being PI, and EX with the territory of being AS.

That stated, if I were to think it appropriate to adjust an IN or an EX as a single (not coupled with another component) listing, I would use a prone thrust on a drop table. These are depicted in the illustration.

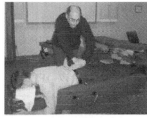 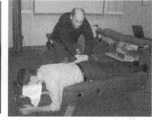

Alternative prone IN drop table move

Alternative prone EX drop table move

Symphysis pubis

Although earlier in this book I made the argument that diastasis of the symphysis pubis is not a very common complaint, despite the fact that the osteopaths are wont to make much of it, it is seen from time to time. The typical patient is most likely to be female, and young at that, and especially recently post-partum. She gave birth a few months ago, sometimes a few years ago, and developed residual

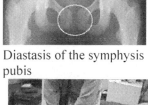

Diastasis of the symphysis pubis

symphysis pain that never resolved, despite reassurement from the ob-gyn or other

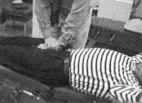

Drop table adjustment of symphysis pubis

doctor. There may have been a referral to a urologist, simply on account of the location of the pain. There are some reports that symphysis dysfunction can produce bladder symptoms, which would amount to somatovisceral reflexes.

Palpating for symphysis subluxation

- Patient locates her open pubic bone
- Pain on side of anterior pube
- Doc replaces patient finger with his or her own
- Replaces palpating finger with pisiform
- Assumes toggle-recoil-like contact
- Thrust 1-3 times

There are two manual treatment methods that are very effective. The first is a drop-table assisted thrust on the symphysis, as seen in the illustration. The adjustment itself is quite straightforward, but getting the hands in place without risking the patient supposing inappropriate contact is something to be carefully considered. I use a procedure that resembles the protocol for performing a toggle recoil adjustment of the atlas.

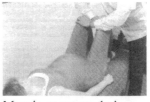

Muscle energy technique for gapping the symphysis. Doctor lets ago suddenly while patient resists bilateral abduction.

The other method for manipulating the symphysis pubis need not be done on a drop table, but is mentioned here for convenience. It is a muscle energy technique, in which the patient's own muscular contraction is deployed to produce gapping and consequent realigning of the symphysis (see illustration, Peterson). The doctor applies a spreading force to the supine patient's flexed knees, while the patient resists. Without warning the doctor lets go, usually producing a cavitation at the symphysis. Although the move is not as vectored as the drop-assisted thrusting procedure, the outcome is very consistently good to excellent.

Months and sometimes years of groin pain can be almost entirely abolished in a millisecond with either of these two excellent adjustive procedures.

Appendix: Patient routing and treatment in a Pierce-Stillwagon technique setting

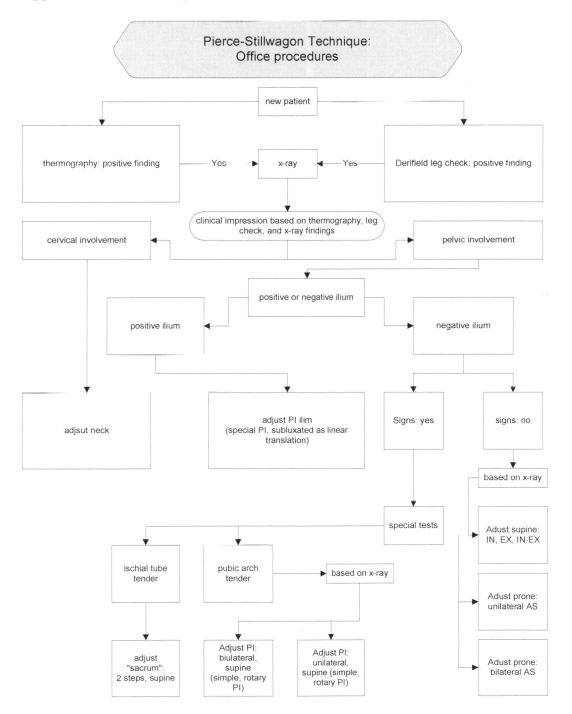

14. Diagnostic and therapeutic blocking[1]

Using padded wedges for lumbopelvic mechanical analysis

Padded wedges, most closely associated with practitioners of Sacro-Occipital Technique[2], are used to treat pelvic torsion. The wedges are placed asymmetrically under the patient, either supine or prone, to serve as fulcrums that allow gravitational forces to affect the position or movement of

Blocking indications
• large patient
• osteoporosis
• previous poor outcome with HVLA
• previous good outcome with blocking
• patient fears cavitation
• SI instability (supine blocking)
• uncertain diagnosis

the sacroiliac and lumbar joints. Blocking may as well be considered an orthopedic test, since the purpose of virtually any such test is to put the joints under investigation in stressed or potentially de-stressed positions, noting the symptomatic changes and drawing the appropriate clinical conclusions. Padded wedges, apart from their value in treating patients, can thus be used to generate diagnostic information as well, that amounts to *mechanically-assisted orthopedic testing.* Following that, it then becomes the doctor's choice as to whether to proceed by adjusting the patient using padded wedges, an HVLA thrust in side posture or on a drop table, a percussive instrument, etc.

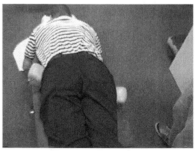

Prone blocking with padded wedges.

The aggravation and/or amelioration of symptoms when joints are stressed into a certain position not only identifies which joints are the worst offenders, but suggests appropriate vectors for treatment. If padded wedges are positioned under the patient so as to increase local symptoms, this is *a priori* evidence that the patient should not be adjusted in this pattern. If padded wedges ameliorate

---

[1] This chapter partially based upon Cooperstein R. Padded wedges for lumbopelvic mechanical analysis. ACA Journal of Chiropractic 2000;37(10):24-26.

[2] Cooperstein R. Technique system overview: Sacro Occipital Technique. Chiropractic Technique 1996;8(3):125-131.

symptoms, an appropriate treatment approach is instantly identified.

It is tempting to conclude that the test results confirm a particular distortion pattern, or movement restriction. For example, the patient shown in the figure, whose pain happens to be ameliorated by the blocking, *may* have a right posterior, left anterior pelvic torsion pattern; or, this patient *may* be restricted in left posterior rotation and/or right anterior innominate rotation; or both. On the other hand, as plausible as these inferences may seem, we need not insist upon them. It is not necessary to go beyond the clinical finding that symptom amelioration speaks in favor of the blocking pattern shown. The treatment options include, but are not limited to, leaving that patient on the blocks for some period of time.

This is may be considered a "black box" approach to treating the patient, based less on a specific mechanical listing, even though some are suggested, and more on our clinical intuition that a pre-adjustive body placement pattern that ameliorates mechanical pain is likely to inform a good clinical outcome, and help avoid aggravation. As all clinicians know, the final examination maneuver – following static and motion palpation, x-ray analysis, leg checks, etc. – is *setting up on the patient.* This "orthopedic test" amounts to a mechanical override switch that prevents us from not seeing the forest for the trees. If the patient winces, tenses up, becomes apprehensive, or even complains as the doctor begins to assert pre-adjustive tension, there is good reason to expect a bad outcome. True, a forceful adjuster may be able to overcome the patient's resistance, but at what price? The best adjustments do not result from the application of irresistible force, but from the doctor finding a way to minimize patient resistance. Diagnostic blocking should be seen as an orthopedic test designed to illuminate the way.

SOT doctors, who pioneered the use of padded wedges, also look for changes in pain severity and location while the patient is on the blocks, but (to my knowledge) in remote locations, like the shoulder girdle, instead of locally, in the sacroiliac and lumbar areas. No doubt they have reasons for doing so, but it seems more clinically intuitive to determine the local effects of blocking procedures. The tender point that will be used to monitor the impact of various blocking vectors may be in the SI joints, the lumbar joints, at the iliolumbar ligament area, in the sacrotuberous ligament, or in any of the musculature. There is no need to overinterpret the exact location of the tender monitoring point, since it will

Diagnostic blocking protocol (thorough)
•   Choose monitoring point   •   4 primary blocking positions   •   double high, double low, 2 diagonal patterns   •   Seek consistent pain provocation patterns   •   Mechanical "diagnosis" actually identifies treatment vectors, not tissue derangement

used less to identify the specific pathology and more the wisdom of alternative treatment vectors.

Theoretically, the blocks may be inserted under the patient in 8 patterns, as can be seen in the table below. Although not strictly required to initiate treatment, and certainly not validated, the table identifies *consistent* positional and movement restriction diagnoses. I am not aware of any evidence that any specific static misalignment of the pelvic bones predicts any specific movement dysfunction pattern. (Where's the chiropractic Rosetta stone when you need it?) Eight patterns is a bit much; in practice, using the so-called "thorough protocol," the blocks are first placed under the patient in the two diagonal patterns (rows 3 and 4 in the table below), and the impact upon the incoming pain complaint assessed. Then, the blocks are placed double high and then double low, corresponding to rows 1 and 2 in the table below, and the pain once again assessed. With all the information logged, the doctor can now design an appropriate treatment: the response to diagonal blocking suggests a possible torsion adjustment (side-posture, drop-table, or blocking), and the response to sagittal plane blocking informs as to whether that adjustive procedure might be best done in flexion, extension, or body neutral positions. Either one move is crafted that satisfies both criteria, or two consistent moves can be performed sequentially. One of the appendices provides an example of how this "thorough protocol" may be used in significantly symptomatic patient, and another appendix shows an alternative "quick scan" that is preferred in a minimally symptomatic or asymptomatic patient.

Blocks may also be inserted under the lumbar spine of the supine patient for diagnostic purposes, a maneuver I sometimes call "Category IV" blocking, in deference to my SOT colleagues who describe Category I, II, and III blocking (1). Lumbar blocking, beyond the scope of this brief article, amounts to a supine version of McKenzie-style pain provocative orthopedic testing (2). Suffice it to say that if blocking in the mid-lumbars reduces lumbopelvic pain, perhaps increasing pain-free straight leg raising and/or well leg raising, then the patient would clinically benefit from the introduction of lumbar extension, through any of a variety of means.

Provocative orthopedic testing using padded wedges

Blocking pattern that ameliorates and/or does not aggravate	Consistent positional inference	Consistent restriction inference
bilateral iliac crests	lumbopelvic hyperextension ("double AS")	restriction in posterior pelvic tilting
bilateral trochanters	lumbopelvic hypolordosis ("double PI")	restriction in anterior pelvic tilting
left crest, right trochanter	left AS / right PI	restriction in left posterior, right anterior innominate rotation
right crest, left trochanter	right AS / left PI	restriction in right posterior, left anterior innominate rotation
left trochanter	left PI	restriction in left anterior innominate rotation
right trochanter	right PI	restriction in right anterior innominate rotation
left iliac crest	left AS	restriction in left posterior innominate rotation
right iliac crest	right AS	restriction in right posterior innominate rotation

Although this chapter has described prone diagnostic blocking, I assume it would also be possible to use the protocol with the patient supine. Although both prone and supine pelvic blocking are intended to reduce pelvic torsion, the mechanics are somewhat different. Prone blocking, by raising the innominate bones relative to the sacrum, distracts the sacroiliac joints; whereas supine blocking, by elevating the innominate bones relative to the sacrum, would be expected to approximate the sacroiliac joints. Whatever the diagnostic findings that accrue to supine blocking maneuvers, the doctor has to decide on clinical grounds whether (apart from reducing the pelvic torsion) the clinical goal is to *mobilize* (prone blocking) or *stabilize* the low back(supine blocking).

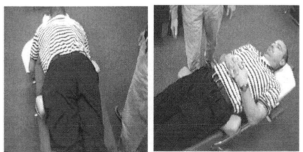

Prone blocking, R-AS, L-PI   Supine blocking, R-AS, L-PI

Using padded wedges for lumbopelvic treatment

The blocks may be used to apply light, gravitationally-assisted forces when place under the patient. The next two figures show supine and prone blocking, respectively, of a patient who exhibits pelvic torsion. The patient exhibits a right-AS/left-PI pattern.

Although both prone and supine pelvic blocking could in principle reduce the pelvic torsion, the mechanics are somewhat different. Prone blocking, by raising the innominate bones relative to the sacrum, would be expected to distract the sacroiliac joints. Supine blocking, by elevating the innominate bones relative to the sacrum would be expected to approximate the sacroiliac joints. The doctor will have to decide whether, in addition to

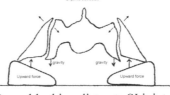 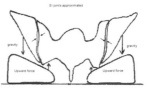

Prone blocking distracts SI joints | Supine blocking approximates SI jts

reducing the pelvic torsion, there is a therapeutic goal of mobilizing (prone preferred) or stabilizing (supine preferred) the sacroiliac joints. The quintessential hypermobile patient is young, female, and pregnant/postpartum.

The figure to the right shows lumbar blocking. It produces relaxation of the low back musculature, primarily quadratus lumborum and sacrospinalis, by approximating their origins and insertions. I am not sure why this sometimes increases straight leg raising, but it may have something to do with inhibiting stretch reflexes that would occur in the low back muscles that would otherwise be provoked by straight leg raising, inhibiting leg raising. By analogy with well-known SOT terminology, ascribing patients to different "categories" depending on which particular style of blocking is appropriate for them, this lumbar blocking may as well be called "Category IV" blocking. It resembles McKenzie-style disk treatment procedures.

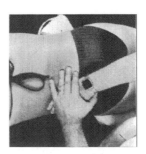

Lumbar blocking

Apart from their use in blocking procedures, the blocks may also be used as fulcrums for HVLA thrusting (see figure). For example, with one or both blocks in position under the prone position, the doctor can "pump" on the sacroiliac joints, by applying mild and repetitive oscillatory thrusts on the PSIS and the ischium, to the contact point not above the block. Or, the doctor may apply a good old-fashioned thrust to one or both of these segmental contact points, with or without drop-table assistance (I think the drop-assisted setup works better). I used to do a move which employed a low block, raising the patient's leg off the table, and adjusting the ipsilateral PSIS on a drop-table (I think I saw this move at a Pettibon seminar. The only patient upon whom I currently perform this is Doctor Vickie, who specifically asks that her right sacroiliac be adjusted in this and no other way.

Although all the blocking situations described so far involve one high and one low block, there are times when the doctor will find it appropriate to insert both blocks high, or both low. Bilateral sub-trochanteric blocking, for example, extends the lumbopelvic area and is of benefit for the same type of patient that benefits from Mackenzie-style extension therapy.

Bilateral ASIS blocking, on the other hand, is of benefit to patients who would benefit more from Cox-style distraction and flexion, especially when employed on the type of table that permits the caudal section underlying the legs to be tilted downward. My Leander table, in my office, has this capability. Bilateral ASIS and trochanteric blocking can also be done supine (not shown) to introduce lumbopelvic extension and flexion, respectively.

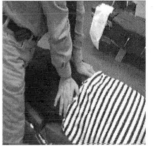 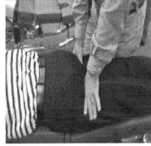

Double PI, prone   Double PI, prone

The chapter on the thoracic spine describes another use of an block, as a fulcrum device for permitted a supine correction of the forward head syndrome, sometimes denoted by the phrase "anterior weight bearing" (AWB). The reader is referred to that chapter for the description of the procedure.

Notes

1.   Cooperstein R. Technique system overview: Sacro Occipital Technique. Chiropractic Technique 1996;8(3):125-131.
2.   McKenzie RA. The lumbar spine: mechanical diagnosis and therapy. Waikanae, New Zealand: Spinal Publications; 1981.
3.   Cooperstein R, Lisi A. Pelvic torsion: anatomical considerations, construct validity, and chiropractic examination procedures. Topics in Clinical Chiropractic 2000;7(3):38-49.

Appendix: The SOT category system

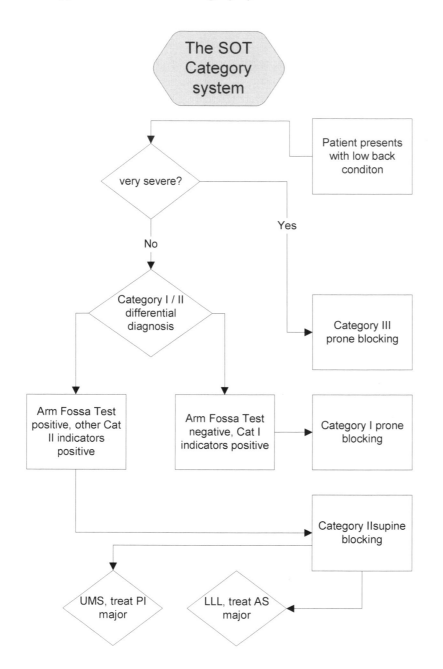

Appendix: quick scan for blocking preferences

Diagnostic blocking protocol (quick scan)

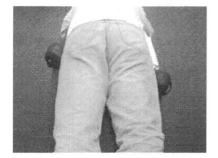

If the left pattern ameliorates while the right pattern aggravates, the patient is a strong responder and the treatment is determinate

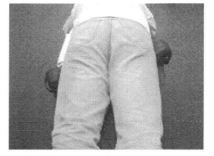

treat for torsion

drop-table, spinal manipulation, blocking, flexion-distraction, instrument adjusting

treat for sagittal plane postural fault

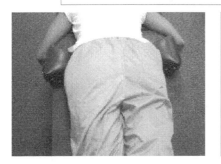

If the left pattern ameliorates while the right pattern aggravates, the patient is a strong responder and the treatment is determinate

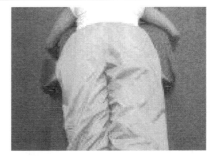

Appendix: Example of deriving adjustive sequence using thorough provocative blocking protocol

Example: Adjustive procedure based on provocative blocking

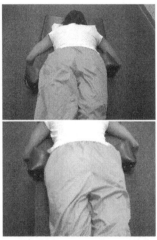
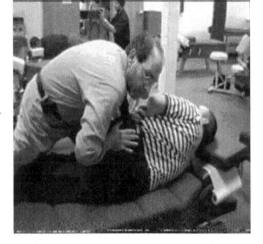

Left PI, in flexion

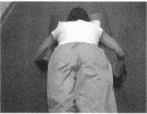
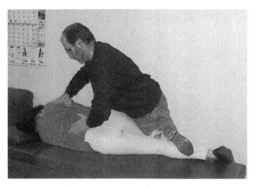

Right PI, in extension

15. Vectored thoracolumbar moves

As we move up in the spine, we get to the thoracolumbar junctional area. Apart from how common it is that patients develop symptoms stemming from this area, often associated with hypertonic, painful fibers in the quadratus lumborum muscles, this is an important region to address even if not currently symptomatic. The fixed point between the mutual, opposed rotations of the shoulder and pelvic girdles during walking is often in this general area, so that movement restriction in this area should be detected when present and corrected. I once had a patient, a tumbler, who complained (among other things) of not being able to tumble straight across the gymnasium on the mats. After being adjusted in the thoracolumbar area, he claimed to now tumble in a truer path, whereupon we agreed, in visits thereafter, that the extent to which he could tumble across the gym in a straight path would be an appropriate outcome measure.

Lumbothoracic junctional region manipulation

It is important to remember that one goal of patient care, including but not restricted to geriatric care, is to assist in maintaining the patient's independence and functional status. Maintaining the integrity of gait and mobility is an essential component of functional status. One of the most characteristic features of the geriatric gait is that the pelvis is carried very stiffly, the legs swung from the hips and the torso failing to participate in ambulation. In more efficient walking, the pelvic and shudder girdles rotate around the Y axis in opposed directions, so that the angular momentum generated by swinging a leg forward is conserved by swinging the opposite arm forward simultaneously. The geriatric patient usually exhibits a hypomobile lumbothoracic junctional area (loosely defined), rendering it difficult for the lumbothoracic spine to participate in the gait mechanism.

This can be seen in the stiff, shuffling gait of the an elderly person. What is particularly insidious about this, from the standpoint of addressing whatever presenting complaints the patient may have, is that the inability to walk in an efficient, comfortable manner without doubt negatively impacts on the value of whatever care is given. Proper walking is necessary for overall biomechanical and psychosocial fitness, and increases the short and long term benefits of adjustive care. Therefore, chiropractic care, whatever the presenting complaints, should include evaluation of the thoracolumbar junction and increasing lumbothoracic mobility, as required.

The kinematics of the lumbothoracic area

As we have discussed previously, we advocate taking the spine's regional kinematic behavior into account in deciding upon an adjustive approach. We have also discussed pre-positioning the patient opposite the presenting distortion, in both the AP and lateral planes, a style ("stress reversal") apparently attributable to Dr. Winterstein of the National College of Chiropractic. Although these considerations are applicable everywhere, the lumbothoracic area provides a particularly interesting opportunity to apply these principles. This can be a challenging area to adjust, not unlike the other transitional areas of the spine, and to get the job done, we could use all the mechanical help we can get.

Adjusting "as if"

As a general rule, spinal manipulation requires less force and achieves quicker and more extensive corrections of postural distortion syndromes when the thrust is applied in accordance with the normal kinematics for the joint concerned. Furthermore, if the patient is pre-positioned by pre-stressing the various joints so as to reverse the presenting distortion, then the manipulative thrust gains access to the paraphysiological space in a manner least likely to incur damage. To put it simply, patients may be pre-positioned to assume the mirror image of their usual distorted posture, and then brought even further toward this "corrected" direction by adjustment in accordance with the normal kinematics for the spinal-pelvic area in question.

Following this method, we find that spinal curvatures can sometimes be influenced in an essentially discontinuous event, rather than requiring a protracted series of "adjustments" that hopefully influence the distortion "just a little bit" at a time. Although there is nothing inherently wrong with promising continuous if not rapid convergence toward less distortion, it would seem preferable to attempt a speedier correction by employing more kinematic principles than are commonly applied. Some postural distortions represent unstable equilibria: small departures from the distortion state are self-limiting and tend to yield rather forthrightly to the return of the original distortion, whereas larger corrective departures seem equipped to traverse the point of no return and suddenly attain a new, qualitatively different equilibrium state featuring a lower potential energy of distortion.

No claim is made that utilizing the principles of kinematic adjusting and vectored pre-positioning guarantees "correction" or even substantial improvement in abnormal curvatures - although sometimes it does. Rather, it is the case that these principles increase the probability that the joints will at minimum be substantially moved, and that soft tissues which have entered into chronic contractures (on the concave sides of abnormal curves) will in fact be lengthened. These methods are preferred to more conventional procedures which call for "torque to close the wedge," an expression referring to the endeavor to reduce the convexity of a lateral curvature of the spine by twisting the wrist of the contact hand, as it were, to somehow spin the segment toward a more proper alignment. If one wishes to "close the wedge," it is easier to bend the patient then to deliver a spinning force of dubious Newtonian significance. Summarizing, whether we realistically expect to effect an improvement in lateral curvature, *we adjust "as if" we could.*

Lovett

Lovett, the early 20th century authority on scoliosis, quotes Bigelow: "The principle of torsion is illustrated by bending a flat blade of grass or a flat, flexible stick in the direction of its width. The center immediately rotates upon its longitudinal axis to bend flatwise in the direction of its thickness. In the same way the spine, laterally flexed, turns upon its vertical axis to yield in its shortest or antero-posterior diameter."[1] Lovett goes on to add, on page 39: "Torsion results from any motion of a straight flexible rod in which all the particles do not move in parallel planes."

The rationale and method of deployment of the thoracolumbar moves herein described devolve directly from the kinematics of spinal coupling patterns. Recalling Lovett, we reiterate that the spine may not accomplish lateral bending without simultaneously performing rotation on its Y axis. This necessity flows directly from the nature of the spine as a flexible rod which is wider in its left-right measurement than it's a-P measurement (functionally speaking). The fact that the spine is segmented and entertains an extensive complex of ligaments and muscles that governs its motions modulates, but does not fundamentally alter, the torsional properties of the spine as a flexible rod.

Coupling patterns of the lumbar spine

When a subject attempts a lateral bend with the thoracolumbar spine in the forward flexed position, the lumbar bodies turn toward the side of the lateral bend; whereas, when a subject attempts a lateral bend with the lumbar spine extended, the opposite occurs, the vertebral bodies rotating opposite the side of bend. Since the subject normally carries the lumbar spine in a lordotic position, the spinous processes therefore generally move toward the concavity of the curve.

---

[1] Lovett RW. Lateral Curvature of the Spine. 4 ed. Philadelphia: P. Blakiston's Son & Co.; 1922 p.20

Haas et al, investigating lumbar spinous process behavior in lateral bending, showed both types of movement commonly occurred.[2]

If a patient were now to present with, say, a left lateral curvature of the lumbar spine, we would like the adjustment to introduce a lateral bend to the left. Given that the spine must rotate (i.e., twist) in order to accomplish this lateral bending, we could conceivably employ either of two strategies: we could turn the vertebral bodies away from the side of bend and then extend the spine, or alternatively, we could turn the vertebral bodies toward the side of bend and complete the motion by flexing the spine a bit. (The reader should confirm that turning his trunk toward the left and flexing forward accomplishes a left lateral lumbothoracic bend, of a sort, as does turning to the right and extending.) We have elected to deploy a strategy for adjusting the lumbothoracic spine based on flexion; it was felt that this would be preferred to an analogous procedure in extension, because this latter would pre-position joints in a more apposed and thus less movable initial state.

Anterior lumbothoracic move

When not contraindicated, our favored manipulative procedure is the "anterior lumbothoracic," modeled after the well-know anterior dorsal maneuver but applied near or below the level of the floating ribs (see below). The patient is sitting on the table with the knees flexed and the feet at the end of the table. This tends to flatten the lumbothoracic lordosis against the table, and also relaxes the psoas muscle which, as an extensor of the spine, could inhibit the desired result. The lower extremities are pre-positioned toward the side of lumbothoracic convexity, and the torso will eventually be lowered toward this same side. (A moment's consideration will confirm that when the legs and the torso are pre-positioned during the adjustment toward the side of the presenting convexity, the lumbothoracic transitional area to be adjusted is placed in an opposite configuration, in the direction of correction.)

Anterior lumbothoracic move

- Synkinetic adjusting
- Adjusting "as if" to correct posture
- Adusting to reduce restriction
- Rule of rights / lefts
- prestress shoulder and pelvic girdles against curvature and/or restriction
- rotate trunk toward prestressed deviations

---

[2] Haas M, Peterson D. A roentgenological evaluation of the relationship between segmental motion and malalignment in lateral bending. Journal of Manipulative and Physiological Therapeutics 1991;15(6):350-360.

The patient's crossed arms are positioned with the elbows overlapping, tucked in very close to the patient's abdomen; this tucked-in position will maintain the lumbothoracic region in flexion when the clinician puts the force in, and furthermore protect the patient from having "the wind knocked out" of him. It will also decrease the pre-thrust apposition of the facetal joints, thereby reducing the force required to obtain further joint separation, and furthermore ensure that the weight of the patient's torso is added to the thrust that is generated by the clinician, thus making for a more effective delivery. The clinician grasps the overlapped elbows with his inferior hand, while placing his superior hand, fingers flexed so that the spinous processes are cradled between the thenar and hypothenar pads. The patient inhales and then exhales as the clinician lowers the torso to the table. As the torso descends, the clinician rolls the shoulders toward the side of leg and torso pre-stress. That is, he or she keeps the torso somewhat more elevated off the table on the side opposite that to which the bending is taking place. This shoulder roll not only facilitates the desired lateral bend, but also unwinds the helical component of the spinal torsion, as described in an earlier chapter. At the moment of the thrust, the doctor's thrusting arm is aimed at the contact hand on the patient's spine, and a line drawn through both would be perpendicular to the table.

Where an HVLA thrust cannot be safely applied, the patient may be gently rocked in the same general position, while the doctor varies the application of the hand behind the spine to mobilize the spinal joints at the various levels. Patients who can not tolerate being supported in the supine position can have their lumbothoracic articulations mobilized in the prone position, but this is not as effective, since this area is built more for flexion than extension, and therefore is best mobilized in flexion. If it must be done prone, a dorsal roll can be placed under the patient's midsection to introduce flexion, or a table that allows lumbopelvic flexion during treatment can be used.

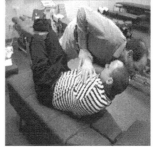

The use of vectored pre-positioning may be employed to adjust the thoracic spine, which generally presents with an area of convexity opposite to that displayed by the lumbar spine of the lumbothoracic transitional area. This is discussed in the next chapter.

Anterior lumbothoracic move.

We need to comment on how the breast tissue, both the doctor's and the patient's, interferes with this move. Some female doctors will have a hard time introducing the force as described, without feeling their chest area has been compromised, whether physically or professionally. Some patients will encounter a similar feeling, since this thrust works best when the doctor's sternal area is applied very closely to the patient's crossed elbows. One way of approaching all this is for the doctor to apply one of their forearms (used thus as a "spacer") across the patient's crossed forearms, and then make contact with their other hand and chest. There are other solutions as well, within the reach of any doctor willing to find a way to get the job done. This is an important move, well worth the trouble to tame.

16. The mid-thoracic spine

The thoracic spine is a transitional relatively hypomobile region between the mobile cervical and lumbar spines. This probably protects the vital organs that are housed within the rib cage, and the rib cage in turn limits the available motion by its system of "hoops." This stabilizing function is lost, incidentally, if the sternum is removed. This same stabilizing function serves to limit the success of postural correction in the thoracic spine as compared with the lumbar spine, given that the architecture of the rib cage locks the chronic deformation in all the more securely. This chapter concerns mostly the mid-thoracic spine, bounded by the thoracolumbar junctional area (discussed in the previous chapter) and the cervicothoracic junctional area (discussed in the next chapter)

Thoracic kinematics

The coupling patterns of the upper thoracic spine are similar to those seen in the cervical spine, in that lateral bending is accompanied by ipsilateral body rotation. Therefore, the spinous processes move toward the convexity of the lateral curve which is formed during a bending motion. However, the coupling pattern in some cases is opposite in the middle thoracic spine, wherein the spinous processes may move toward the concavity of the curve that is formed (behaving like lumbar vertebrae). Grieve says that the upper thoracic spine behaves much like the cervical spine, and the lower thoracic spine much like the lumbar spine, while the portion in-between may need "to make its mind up."[1] Grieve says that in the thoracic and lumbar spines, side flexion is accompanied by body rotation to the same side only if the subject is in forward flexion simultaneously, and occurs oppositely if the subject is extended. These findings are completely consistent with the finding of Lovett, whose pioneering work was done early in the twentieth century, discussed in the previous chapter.

We should point out that Haas[2] found that movement of the lumbar spinous processes *away from* the side of lateral bending was very common, occurring in

---

[1] Grieve G. Common Vertebral Joint Problems. 1 ed. Edinburgh London Melbourne and New York: Churchill Livingstone; 1981, p. 96

[2] Haas M, Peterson D. A roentgenological evaluation of the relationship between segmental motion and malalignment in lateral bending. Journal of Manipulative and Physiological Therapeutics 1991;15(6):350-360.

about 1/3 if his subjects. He felt this "type II" spinous behavior was so common that it should be considered a normal variant, and we would imagine this finding could extend into the lower thoracic spine as well. Whatever happens when a subject bends to the side, we would at least expect left-right symmetry, lacking which we presume a dysfunctional state worthy of attention.

The thoracolumbar junctional area has been stated to be a mortise joint, wherein flexion movements are more important than extension movements. This is also the most commonly injured area of the thoracic spine. We addressed this area in the previous chapter. The cervicothoracic junctional area is functionally part of the neck, and is mostly described from a treatment point of view in the next chapter, although the assessment part is best described in this chapter.

Assessment of the thoracic spine

Our discussion here, as it logically should, will resemble what we have said previously about the lumbar spine. There are both global and local parameters, as always, to take into account. Globally, we identify both lateral curvatures of the spine, and asymmetries in lateral bending behavior. We could also look for differences in rotational behavior, but to my knowledge there is nothing published on this except for range of motion information, which does not really lead to much in terms of knowing where or how to adjust, as of this time. Locally, we look for segmental restrictions, misalignments, and soft tissue textural changes. Although the paragraphs immediately below concern *assessment*, the temptation to jump to the implications for adjustive strategies is irresistible, and thus some of this shows up in these same paragraphs.

Thoracic spine appearance and palpation

Lateral curvature: scoliosis

The thoracolumbar spine often forms an s-shaped scoliosis, with the lumbar portion convex on the side of the posterior innominate cleavage, and the thoracic spine convex on the opposite side. In cases where the lumbar spine is hard to visualize or palpate, it may be easier to infer its structure from the more easily discerned structure of the thoracic spine. Obviously, it is always better to palpate the lumbar spine as compared with inferring anything about its structure, but we must remember to always be realistic: if the palpatory procedure is of questionable reproducibility, and the evidence is not overwhelming anyway, then one would have more confidence in predicting the lumbar spine from a very clear read on the thoracic spine.

Given that the thoracic spine may exhibit more superiorly a second curvature opposite in its direction from its first curvature, it is important that the examiner ascertain that she or he has truly detected the first thoracic compensation to the lumbar convexity. These curvatures can be palpated, and can also be directly visualized in which case the task is made easier if the spinous processes are marked with a wax pencil. As discussed above, the identification of thoracic lateral curvature is likely to affect the line of drive, once the decision to intervene has been made on clinical grounds.

We could get far astray by getting too heavily involved in discussion of scoliosis, both the cases of idiopathic juvenile scoliosis and more physiological curvatures of the spine. We have already taken the opportunity to comment that when confronted with lateral curvature, we emphasize adjustive strategies that are directed into the convexity, "as if" we could straighten the curvature. Again, we would not turn down any lessening of the curvature, unless, of course, it were associated with the patient (remember him?) feeling worse, but our *goal is less to straighten the spine and more to optimize the intervention.*

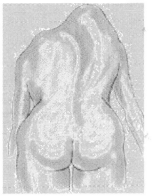

Note Adam's sign.

Is this straight spine the only possible "normal" spine structure?

Thoracic lateral curvature is easier to see than lumbar curvature, but if there is any doubt about it, we simply have the patient flex at the waist and look for posterior humping: the Adam's sign. In addition, we note that thoracic spinal convexity is often associated with winging of the ipsilateral scapula, 70% of the time according to one authority (Schafer, R.C.). These lateral curvatures can be assessed in the prone position as well, but usually the magnitude is diminished, and more rarely, the curvature disappears or even reverses.

Apart from noting the presence or absence of spinal lateral curvatures, we are quite curious as to how they behave in lateral bending activities, as discussed below. There is good reason to believe that the kinematics of the scoliotic spine, its *dynamics*, are very similar to those of the more or less straight spine, in terms of where the spinous processes go during lateral bends. From the standpoint of *statics*, we generally find the spinous process have gone to the concavity when there is long-standing curvature of the spine.

Segmental thoracic analysis

As always, segmental analysis involves the identification of misalignment, restricted movement, soft tissue textural changes, etc. We have little to add here to what has been discussed in the introductory chapters, as well as in the chapter on the lumbar spine. This is not surprising: the thoracic and lumbar spinal joints present the same examination questions for the prone patient. We have seen at least one segmental problem in the thoracic spine frequently, not occurring much in the lumbar spine, that we have taken the liberty of terming "tortithoracis." This is described below, in the part of the chapter dealing with treatment approaches.

Static and dynamic analysis: congruent or divergent?

There would be no problem if a person with a right thoracic convexity were restricted in right lateral bending. In such a case a thrust from right to left, directed so as to "close the wedge" (as one popular chiropractic technique would put it) would correct both the positional fault and the motion restriction. Indeed, it is commonly believed that impaired lateral flexion to the right *results from* a segmental convexity on the right, so that a static listing may be inferred from motion findings. A doctor often claims a "PLS" at T6 purely on the basis of impaired bending to the right, perhaps without any other radiological or static palpatory information in support of that diagnosis. (We are not certain if the same argument is made regionally, so that right lateral curvature would be said to predict globally restricted right lateral flexion.)

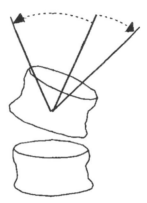

The left open wedge is associated with *increased* lateral bending to the left, assessed from the start point. This opposes what is commonly believed. (Adapted from Haas.)

Unfortunately, this belief may be unwarranted. Haas showed that the direction of lateral flexion malposition does indeed predict motion asymmetry, but in a manner opposite to what has been commonly believed[3] (see right figure). That is, the PLS described above will usually be associated with increased motion to the left! Now, this is not a pretty thing, amounting to yet another beautiful theory slain by an ugly fact.

Nonetheless, like any other study, it should be replicated before one draws radical conclusions from it. The authors themselves indicate that the precise interpretation of their findings depends to some degree on how the lateral flexion malposition is measured. Furthermore, it is not clear whether the mechanical tendencies they describe for segmental lesions may be directly extrapolated to more regional analyses of spinal behavior; that is, might a spinal region behave in

---

[3] Haas M, Peterson D. A roentgenological evaluation of the relationship between segmental motion and malalignment in lateral bending. Journal of Manipulative and Physiological Therapeutics 1991;15(6):350-360.

accordance with the conventional wisdom, even if individual motion segments do not? In any case, a strong case is made for strongly reconsidering the classic motion palpation "rule" that restricted lateral flexion to a given side indicates an "open wedge" on that side at that spinal segment.

Returning to the problem at hand, we note that the criteria provided by static analysis and dynamic analysis could lead us in different directions, in terms of an adjustive strategy. We can no longer assume that an open wedge correlates with reduced lateral bending, and therefore that one and the same thrust is likely to improve both situations. If there is no clear preponderance of evidence pointing toward either the static lateral curvature or dynamic lateral bending analysis as of greater significance, my convention is to favor the dynamic analysis. Indeed, there appears to be a developing profession-wide consensus that the motion properties of the spine should take priority over the static findings. On the other hand, if the patient has very noticeable lateral curvature, the temptation to try to reduce it is virtually irresistible, at least for me.

Motion palpation studies have tended not to show very good reliability in the thoracic spine. In our own study, we were able to achieve a high level of concordance by changing the methodology in two ways: first, we used continuous analysis, amenable to ICC and rather the Kappa statistic; and second, we used confidence calls. The method we used involved assessing for endfeel, rather than excursion.

The sagittal thoracic curves

There is probably (at least I think) lots of agreement among clinicians that abnormal sagittal curves are more problematic than lateral curvatures in the frontal plane. The thoracic curve, which may, in a functional sense, extend into the lower cervical spine or the upper lumbar spine, should be kyphotic. Although the evidence on what constitutes a "normal" amount and shape of thoracic kyphosis, is spotty, notwithstanding the suggestions of Drs. Pettibon and Harrison, at least at the extremes there would be little disagreement among clinicians that too much kyphosis or too little kyphosis could pose a problem.

Forward head with thoracic hyperkyphosis.

Exaggerated upper dorsal kyphosis is often associated with forward head syndrome (aka: round shoulders, anterior weight bearing, etc.), and is better discussed in the context of treatment, below. For the moment, let us say that the patient describes pain in the "shoulders," often accompanied by chronic tension headaches and pain in the back of the arms. There may be tingling in the fingers and other problems commonly described as part of the thoracic outlet syndrome. The worst cases, of course, result from a Gibbus deformity, but these cases and the Dowager's hump occur only infrequently in relation to the more garden variety cases of stooped shoulders that chiropractors treat. I describe my favored manipulative approach to this problem in the next chapter, under the heading "anterior weight bearing move."

Exaggerated mid and lower thoracic kyphosis is sometimes associated with Scheuermann's juvenile kyphosis, amounting to a post-traumatic sequela. Afflicted individuals manifest much rigidity and do experience chronic dorsal pain. When not associated with a Scheurmann's-type situation, thoracic hyperkyphosis is often related to a full-body postural distortion, whether lumbar hyperlordosis, sway-back (linear translation of the pelvis anteriorly), or the flat-back posture (all the sagittal curves are reduced and the head is displaced anteriorly). Any attempt at ameliorating the thoracic hyperkyphosis should be linked to a full-body postural improvement strategy.

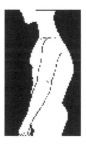

Thoracic hypokyphosis often occurs in the mid to upper dorsals, where it is commonly described as "saucering" or as "Pottenger's saucer." It is strongly related to the patient complaint of "pain between the shoulder blades." These are difficult cases to treat. The obvious goal of care is to improve the kyphosis, but in fact, we generally have to settle for not worsening the problem, by not thrusting P to A into the already-hyperextended thoracic spine. The more appropriate anterior thoracic adjustment is discussed below.

Analysis of lateral flexion

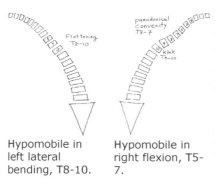

Hypomobile in left lateral bending, T8-10.

Hypomobile in right flexion, T5-7.

Let us begin with an apparently "normal" spine that is reasonably straight in the frontal plane. The caption in the right figure suggests there is plenty of room for discussion as to what "normal" is. Some authorities, including Gray's Anatomy and Kendall and McCreary, have suggested that there is a relationship between handedness and spinal curvatures, such that it would be normal for a right-handed individual to exhibit a right convex thoracic curve, and a left-handed individual a left convex thoracic curve. The more fundamental question raised is, even given that frontal plane curvatures may be "normal" and related to other neural (left/right brain) and visceral asymmetries that are "hard-wired" into the body's structure, whether such curvatures sooner or later lead to mechanical breakdown and patient complaints.

In any case, whatever "normal" is, when a patient is passively flexed to the side, we would expect the spine to describe a smooth arc, in which no segments make a significantly smaller or greater contribution to the overall arc than any of the others. Essentially, this is my preferred method for conducting "motion palpation" of the thoracic (and lumbar) spines, a sort of hybrid of dynamic and static methods.

However, it can be seen in the figure that in right lateral bending, segments T5-T7 remains somewhat convex to the right, indicating spinal hypomobility in that region in right lateral bending. I commonly use the terms "flattened" and "paradoxically convex" to describe such hypomobilities. These terms indicate a failure to fully participate, or an actually bucking of the trend, respectively. Not surprisingly, there is a hypermobile spinal unit at T9-10, manifested by the kink that can be see in the arc at this point. By "kink" I mean a local discontinuity in the curve, an interruption of the smoothness of the arc.

Most chiropractors would agree that there would be some value in applying a force at the clearly hypomobile region, at T5-7, directed so as to increase lateral flexion to the right (as discussed below), but there would be more controversy on the wisdom of applying a force to the T9-10 spinal unit. After all, isn't it written that "thou shalt not adjust a hypermobile segment"? Although not oblivious to this commandment, it needs a qualifier: "thou shalt not adjust a hypermobile segment so as to increase the motion in the direction into which its motion is excessive."

The same spine could show very different behavior in lateral bending to the right, as in the figure to the right. Here, there is a hypomobile region at T8-10, manifested by flattening in this region during left lateral flexion, a failure to participate in the bend. The assumption is that it would be a priori reasonable to apply a thrust that increased motion in the direction of hypomobility, granted that it is contraindicated to thrust in the opposite direction, at least in this example. It would be beneficial if discussion were cast in terms of the hypomobile direction, and not so much the hypomobile "segment."

So far, we have explored the lateral bending behavior of a straight spine. What if the subject starts out with lateral curvature, as in the figure below, in which the subject starts lateral bending from an initial position of large right thoracic curvature, and mild left lumbar curvature.

When there are initial lateral curvatures of the thoracic spine, nothing fundamental changes in the dynamic assessment of motion, as described above. The patient is flexed to the right and to the left, while the examiner detects spinal kinks, flattened, and paradoxically convex regions and motion segments. In this example, the right lumbar curve corrects, suggesting it is functional, but the left thoracic curvature persists, suggesting it is structural, and worthy of more treatment.

As discussed below (see "Static and dynamic analysis: congruent or divergent?"), when static malpositions (lateral curvatures) are present, this raises the possibility of an incompatibility between classic "sticky joint" and "crooked bone" types of criteria for determining segmental contact points and line of correction. Starting from a static well-aligned spine, we need only worry about dynamic dysfunction; but starting from a spine with significant lateral curvature, there is no guarantee that what we might choose to do from a static point of view will be optimal from a dynamic point of view.

Sometimes the terms "primary" and "secondary" are used to make the same distinction, but I avoid them because these same terms are used to distinguish congenital and developmental sagittal curves; e.g., the "primary" dorsal kyphosis, and the "secondary" cervical lordosis. Chiropractors have also used the word "compensation" to indicate a curvature which is functional and adaptive.

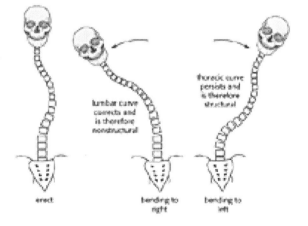

These findings indicate a clinical strategy, in that the structural lateral curvatures warrant more attention than the functional lateral curvatures. In practice, this means I will manipulate obvious structural curvatures on most office visits, whereas the functional, compensatory curvatures would receive attention less frequently.

Adjustive strategies

Adjusting the thoracic lateral curvature

The use of vectored pre-positioning may be employed to adjust the thoracic spine, which generally presents with an area of convexity opposite to that displayed by the lumbar spine of the lumbothoracic transitional area. The maneuver is exactly the same as what was described in the chapter on the vectored lumbothoracic adjustment, except this time there is no need to keep the knees bent. Furthermore, there is no need to employ shoulder roll, insofar as there is too much inherent variability among individuals in the thoracic kinematics to predict the optimal direction. The rule is: deviate the legs and the trunk of the supine patient toward the convex side of the original presenting thoracic lateral curvature, then put the force in.

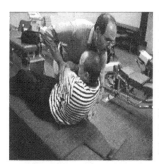

Anterior thoracic maneuver.

In patients who present with thoracic hyperkyphosis, there is still a role for prepositioning, except the adjustment is performed with the patient in the prone position. The same strategy of pre-positioning the legs and the trunk toward the side of the lateral curvature is employed. It may be necessary to allow the patient to turn the head, to either side, whatever is more comfortable for the patient.

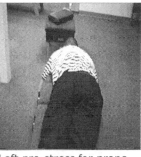

Left pre-stress for prone correction of left thoracic lateral curvature.

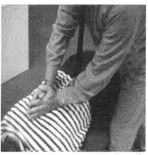

Use of Carver bridge for pre-stressed thoracic posterior adjustment.

A note on "closing the wedge"

Many chiropractors attempt to reduce lateral curvature of the spine in our adjustments by "torquing down the spine to close the wedge." Perhaps it would not be altogether unreasonable to suggest that the most efficient way of closing the wedge would be *to close the wedge!* (We have already made a similar point in the chapter on the vectored lumbothoracic protocol.) That is, the prone or supine patient could be prestressed toward correction prior to the administration of the thrust. Then, the doctor need only deliver his or her best thrust in a linear fashion, without needing to rotate the contact hand around the longitudinal axis of the forearm.

Thus, prestressing the patient as described takes the place of applying torque to "close" or "open" wedges, as the phrase goes. The concept of torque has not fared well in recent years, ranging from theoretical claims to the effect that the vectors applied cannot possibly achieve the stated goals, to laboratory studies purporting to show that such attempts result merely in tugging the skin. On the other hand, laterally flexing the patient so as to reverse the lateral curvature, prior to applying a P to A or an A to P thrust, achieves the stated purpose in a far more intuitive manner. At the least, irrespective of whether there is any lasting alteration in the lateral curvature, the cavitation event is easier to achieve when the deck has been stacked, so to speak, in favor of "correction." Again, we adjust "as if" we could correct things, and indeed, sometimes we can.

Classical chiropractic has largely emphasized "closing the wedge," that is, thrusting into the convex side of spinal lateral curvatures, some believing the pathological entity to consist in subluxation of discal elements toward this side of convexity, and the corrective thrust as repositioning the displaced elements of the intervertebral disk. Physical therapists, osteopaths, and others have generally tended to see the primary lesion to consist in soft-tissue contractures on the concave side of the spinal lateral curvature. The chiropractic orthopedist Stonebrink has developed a theory and practice built upon a parallel concept, wherein distraction of shortened tissues is the primary goal of manipulative therapy.

Indeed, it seems more people these days emphasize opening the closed wedge compared with closing the open wedge. With lateral curvature, it seems that the disc spaces remain relatively normal on the misidentified "open" side of the wedge, whereas the disc spaces are reduced on the correctly identified "closed" side of the wedge. Many of the manipulative and other procedures I perform are explicitly designed to elongate shortened tissue. A good example of this is the distractive maneuver for the atlanto-occipital joint, described in the cervical chapter below.

Adjusting for exaggerated and diminished kyphosis

If a patient appears to be hyperkyphotic, the most optimal forces are P to A. On the other hand, if a patient appears to be saucered (hypokyphotic), it will be more strategic to apply A to P forces. This is because the doctor always has the option, in performing the anterior thoracic maneuver, of keeping the patient's torso off the table at the moment the thrust is delivered. This has the mechanical effect of repositioning the patient's spine in flexion, which reverses the presenting hypokyphosis. It also has the effect of reducing the apposition of the thoracic facets, which facilitates the gapping and sheering that result from the manipulative thrust.

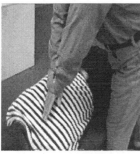 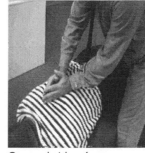 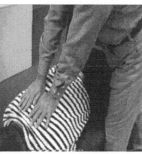

Single-hand contact applies force unilaterally

Carver bridge (very ergonomic).

Double thenar (less ergonomic)

Thoracic hyperkyphosis

The common sense approach to exaggerated kyphosis is a P to A thrust on the prone patient. We have already gone into this to same extent, in our discussion above of methods to reduce lateral curvature. The various traditional contacts include the double thenar, single-hand contact (transverse process contact preferred by patients to spinous process contact), Carver bridge, and crossed pisiform (see figure below). I have little reason to suppose any of these contacts has any therapeutic advantage over another, although there are some differences form an ergonomic point of view. The double thenar contact, used over and over, may eventually result in a wrist sprain, which then heals slowly due to the likelihood of additional trauma as the doctor continues to adjust patients. At the other end of the ergonomic spectrum is the Carver bridge, which possesses the same advantage as keyboards that are designed to protect the typist's wrist by keeping the hands partially supinated.

When the kyphosis is the result of Scheurmann's disease, compression fractures, inflammatory arthritis, or congenital malformation, all bets are off; it is difficult to predict the results in treating such cases with manipulation, prone or supine. Among those patients who do benefit from manipulation, A to P maneuvers are often better tolerated, even though on strict mechanical grounds the P to A thrust might seem more optimal.

Diminished thoracic kyphosis

As for diminished kyphosis, one cringes at the thought of battering the spine P to A, for obvious mechanical reasons. Many of the chiropractors who deploy the "anterior thoracic" move, applied A to P on the supine patient, recommend applying this maneuver to the caudad segment of the saucered region of the spine. There, they suggest, one encounters a hyperflexion malposition, compensating for the more cephalad vertebra that would by fixated in hyperextension (hypokyphosis).

I am not sure about the mechanical reasoning here, but at any rate, I do not see the anterior thoracic adjustment as really being "A to P" as compared with P to A thoracic adjustments. The fulcrum under the supine patient introduces local extension when the thrust is delivered through the rib cage, not obviously different from the local extension introduced by a P to A thrust on a prone patient. The difference is that the doctor can easily deliver the anterior thoracic adjustment with the patient positioned with the trunk flexed off the table. In other words, the mechanical approach to the patient who has lost, in effect, thoracic flexion is to adjust the patient in flexion. Summarizing, the underlying mechanics are probably more or less the same in thoracic posteriors and anteriors; the primary difference is how we define the "force" and the "resistance." One supposes Newton could care less.

The anterior thoracic adjustment works best when the doctor does not so much thrust into the patient's crossed forearms, as *squeeze the patient against the table* to the point of implosion, prior to applying an abrupt body drop as the doctor's cephalad knee buckles. I prefer the variation of the move in which the doctor's superior hand is under the patient, to the approach in which the doctor's inferior hand reaches around to be placed underneath the patient. This latter approach works well for relatively small patients, but unless the doctor happens to have orangutang-length arms, the former approach is more likely to be suited *for all patients*. In addition, unless the patient is very heavy, I do *not* support the anterior thoracic approach in which the fully supine patient is slightly rolled to allow the doctor's hand to gain access to the spine; this precludes adjusting the patient in flexion, one of the major advantages of the protocol under discussion.

Adjusting to address lateral flexion restriction

Having performed a sitting lateral flexion test, to visualize and palpate the degree to which the various mid-thoracic levels are participating in lateral bending, one can then determine whether pre-stress in the left or right-bent position is indicated. A similar decision is also made in regards to lateral curvature. Ideally, the criteria for pre-stress to either the left or right, whether in the prone or supine positions, are consistent. In other words, a person who has a left convex region also has restriction in left lateral bending, and vice versa. For each criterion, the one dynamic and the other static, the indication is for pre-stress in left bending. What happens in the case of paradoxical criteria, where dynamic analysis leads to left pre-stress and static analysis to right pre-stress? Then, we will have to weight the findings by clinical severity. For example, if the lateral bending asymmetry is obvious and quantitatively significant, whereas the lateral curvature is barely present or not very clinically impressive, then we will have to go with the dynamic finding to determine our direction of pre-stress. The opposite state of affairs would mandate emphasizing the static findings.

Tortithoracis[4]

Tortithoracis is a made-up word, made up by me. I had learned the word *torticollis* during my undergraduate chiropractic studies, and later learned the term *tortipelvis* from Dr. Barge's books, which I read with great enthusiasm. (I thought he had coined the term, but later found it in the orthopedic medicine literature from decades past.)

In acute tortithoracis, the patient walks in with a "poker spine," and sits very erect on the edge of the chair, or on the examination table. He or she breathes very shallowly, and reports a sharp pain that radiates from the spine following the course of the ribs. The pain becomes worse when he attempts to take a deep breath. Coughing, sneezing, and other sudden motions aggravate the lancinating, very specifically located pain, generally just on the articular pillar, either unilaterally or bilaterally. The pain began while swimming, reaching for an object on a high shelf, working in an awkward position under a car, or while climbing a rope during a difficult weekend serving in the military reserve. These are typical patients.

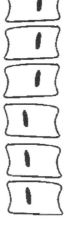

Physical examination reveals a more or less linear offset of a row of spinous processes, as shown in the figure. (which also shows the segmental contact points for the prone correction, as discussed below). The radiating costal pain is usually maximal on the side to which the cephalad spinous processes deviate. It can be determined by palpation of the transverse processes that the segmental discontinuity is essentially rotatory in nature, although in some cases there may be a small element of lateralisthesis as well.

Tortithoracis also presents as a chronic condition as well, in which the spinous process offset is similar, but the pain is less severe and there is no discomfort in deep breathing. No doubt in some offices this same patient would be found to have a "rib head" out or maybe intercostal neuralgia, but I believe tortithoracis to be more an inclusive musculoskeletal complex involving the costovertebral, costotransverse, and intervertebral facetal joints.

---

[4] This discussion of tortithoracis is based on an article published in Dynamic Chiropractic, which itself was based on the discussion in an earlier edition of Chiropraxis.

It is very useful to mark the spinous processes with the letter "X" and clearly observe the offset by sighting the spine longitudinally from either the head or foot of the table (see figure 2).

Following the adjustment I am about to describe, post-check by marking the spinous processes with the letter "O", so as to confirm reduction of the misalignment. It is not uncommon to find that the preadjustive "X" marks have deviated as much as ½ inch from their previous positions, usually in the region cephalad to the former misalignment.

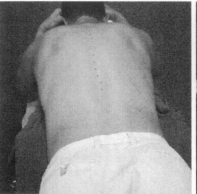 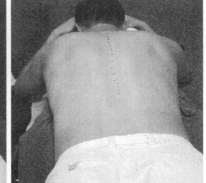

Use water-soluble ink to mark spinous processes pre-adjustment.

Post-adjusment spinous process marking

We treat acute tortithoracis with a single anterior thoracic maneuver, contact hand right on the discontinuity. Relief is very sudden, and very complete. The main difficulty the doctor experiences is avoiding being put off by the intensity of the patient's pain and fear. I see no role for ice, massage, trigger point work, stretching, or any of the shake'n'bake modalities prior to delivering the adjustment. Later on, the accompanying myofascitis can be treated as the doctor sees fit. Chances are the problem will return, whether within a week or a year, because ligaments have stretched and the spinal articulations have become unstable. This will require long run rehabilitation through strengthening the trunk muscles.

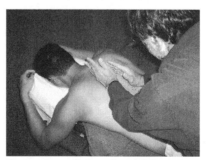

Chronic tortithoracis tends to respond better, for whatever reason, to a P to A thrust. The particular setup I use is borrowed from an Applied Kinesiology text[5], where it is purported to treat "fixations" as compared with "subluxations." (I make no such claim.) For me, this unusual contact existed for many years as an interesting

Correction of chronic tortithoracis

mechanical maneuver awaiting an appropriate condition for which it could be used. (Enter tortithoracis.) The doctor's two hands each contact a different vertebra on the prone patient, one on either side of the spine, according to the rotational parameters of the subluxated joint. The black circles in the figure above

---

[5] Walther DS. Applied Kinesiology, Volume I. Pueblo, Colorado: Systems DC; 1981.

indicate the segmental contact points for this prone adjustment. I generally use a Carver bridge, making sure to stagger the pisiform contacts far enough apart to make sure that they are on different vertebrae.

Torticollis, tortithoracis, tortipelvis. It would appear the cycle is complete . . . unless, well, would you believe torticranium? I remember the entity "banana head" from my studies of craniopathy a long time ago. Will that do, or will someone have to find a better clinical entity to correspond to torticranium?

17. The cervicothoracic junctional area

We have mentioned from time to time the postural aberration that commonly occurs in this region, called forward head syndrome in medicine and often anterior weight bearing in chiropractic, and round shoulders by the man or woman on the street. In addition to this sagittal plane problem, the cervicothoracic junctional area often runs into problems in the frontal plane by attempting to compensate for lateral curvatures in the thoracic and/or lumbar spines. Moreover, it may also attempt to atone for lateral curvatures in the upper and lower cervical spine regions. Like transitional areas in general, if often becomes rather restricted, especially when the patient has anterior weight bearing of the head and neck relative to the trunk. Cruelly, it can be just as difficult for the chiropractor to adjust as it is for the patient to carry around in a state of subluxation.

Cervicothoracic assessment procedures

We have already described manual methods to determine segmental restriction (let us recall our emphasis on quality, over quantity, of movement available). Nothing changes here, nothing to add to the subject of segmental evaluation. From a regional point of view, however, it turns out that the cervicothoracic area is particularly amenable to the use of objective measurement of the range of motion. We must stipulate that some of what passes for "cervical" range of motion includes the participation of the upper thoracic spine, which is why these methods are discussed in this chapter rather than the next.

Inclinometry and goniometry

There are several devices available for measuring the active and passive range of motion for the cervical spine. Some systems are computerized, whereas the others use some sort of protractor or hinged angle-finder. A very effective and inexpensive device called an *inclinometer* is available at most hardware and building supplies stores. It has proven to be very easy and convenient to use to assess lateral and forward flexion, as well as extension. We use an angle goniometer for the assessment of rotation.

Inexpensive, handheld inclinometer.

Inclinometric methodology

The subject sits on an examination bench, and may be asked to grip the underside of the bench with his or her hands to stabilize the torso (this method recommended by Nansel et al.[1] I say "may be asked to grip" bench, because at the current time I am more likely not to do so. I have noticed that when the patient grips the underside of the table to stabilize his or her torso during the inclinometric examination, it may influence the degree of lateral bending. Some patients manifest an increase, and others a decrease, in their active range of motion when their hands grip. It is not at all clear what the underlying biomechanical rationale is for this effect, nor is it clear whether it needs to be addressed to interpret the information provided. As an alternative to having the patient grip the table, the doctor may simply do his or her best to take a reading at the end of lateral flexion just as the unstabilized patient's torso begins to move, or using a second goniometer affixed to the patient's posterior thorax, when the torso has moved no more than a predetermined limit, say 2 degrees.

Proceeding with our description of the goniometric method, the patient's eyes are closed, and the patient is allowed to "warm up" a little with one circumduction in each direction. After zeroing the inclinometer on the vertex of the skull, the examiner measures the excursion of lateral flexion to each side. Great care is taken to avoid extraneous rotation of the head and neck, so that the excursion takes place in one frontal plane. Indeed, when a patient can not avoid taking the head and neck out of plane during an attempted pure lateral flexion, the astute observer already knows which are the offending tissues. For example, suppose a patient extends slightly as his head is conducted to the right. That implies that he is willing to stretch the *anterior* cervical tissues on the left, as need be, to simulate a normal degree of right lateral flexion, but is most cautious about stretching the *posterior* tissues on the left. Those doctors who can read unconscious patient body language surely possess an insight denied to those who can not.

Multiple measures are taken, approximately 3 per side. Generally there is a mild increase in the passive range of motion, so that the 3rd call tends to be the value that is recorded. It should be noted that in the case of torticollis, discussed below, the subject will be virtually incapable of any lateral flexion towards the side of pain, likewise rotation toward the side of pain.

The inclinometer may also be used to measure forward flexion and extension. Extension is markedly limited in cases of cervicobrachialgia, that is, arm pain

---

[1]Nansel DD, Peneff AL, Jansen RD, Cooperstein R. Interexaminer concordance in detecting joint-play reliability with respect to the detection of joint-play asymmetries in the cervical spines of otherwise asymptomatic subjects. Journal of Manipulative and Physiological Therapeutics 1989;12(6):428-433.

and/or numbness related to cervical DJD. Having measured lateral and forward flexion and extension, we next obtain measurements for rotation. Some authorities recommend using the inclinometer with the subject supine, by placing it on the forehead, but we prefer using an angle inclinometer on the top of the patient's skull, because it is weight-bearing and more relevant to the patient's daily life. This requires standing on the table or a chair behind the patient, and some experience in knowing where to place the pivot of the instrument, but one does one's best.

Interpretation of gross patterns

We see two primary patterns of asymmetry emerge. In the first, which is the most common pattern, lateral flexion reduction and rotation reduction are *contralateral*. The simplest explanation is that the posterior cervicodorsal tissues, let's say on the right, limit both lateral flexion to the left and rotation to the right. When overpressure is applied in lateral flexion, the patient usually complains of pain in the upper cervical tissues

Diff-Di: Upper cervical vs. cervicothoraic problem
•   Check lateral flexion and rotation of head-neck
•   Patterns:
•   Ipsilateral restriction: upper cervical rotational subluxation, sub-clinical torticollis, supraclavicular tender nodule opposite pain side
•   Contralateral restriction: cervicothoracis subluxation, hypertonic post trap opp pain side
•   Check for out-of-plane lateral flexion

opposite the side of bend. I do not interpret that to mean there is an upper cervical subluxation or other lesion, but rather that there is soft tissue tethering that puts the brake on lateral flexion, that is experienced mostly in the upper cervical attachment areas. The overall treatment might include soft tissue work on these tethering tissues, although a nice thrust that stretches these tissues abruptly often suffices to get the job done without any additional need for explicit soft tissue work. We sometimes so emphasize the osseous impact of thrusting procedures that we neglect their impact on the soft tissues that attach to bone.

Less commonly, perhaps one-third of the time, overpressure results in pain *ipsilateral* to the side of lateral flexion reduction, and the patient identifies a very focal point of maximum pain in the cervicodorsal region. This point can be confirmed by compression testing, prestressed in various positions as need be. I believe this generally identifies an articular structure as the offender, rather than tethering soft tissue. It will be adjusted, as such.

In the second gross pattern of cervicodorsal limitation, one finds lateral flexion reduction and rotation reduction that is *ipsilateral*. This is considerably less common, perhaps 15 percent of cases. The patient simply does not want to bend or rotate to the same side. Since these are the same motion findings that would be found in torticollis, although not as severe as in the latter case, it would be fair to call this pattern "subclinical toritcollis." It can not be called "torticollis," by definition, since the head and neck is not kept in a cock-robin position; but it surely related. The problem generally turns out to be a significant rotational malalignment in the upper cervical spine, and is treated accordingly. We discuss torticollis a little further below, which presents some obvious problems from a manipulative point of view.

Cervicothoracic manipulative procedures

Anterior weight bearing (AWB) protocol

When the center of gravity of the patient's head is displaced anteriorly relative to the rib cage, it increases the amount of work that the upper dorsal and posterior cervical muscles must perform in order to balance the cranium on the lateral masses of the atlas. This predisposes to upper dorsal fibrosis, tension headaches, thoracic outlet

> Anterior weight bearing (AWB)
>
> - When segmental analysis just won't do . . .
> - prone T2 drop uncomfortable
> - stretch pectorals
> - take broad contact
> - sharp thrust, LOD above block
> - respect contraindications!
> - osteoporosis
> - shoulder girdle instability

syndromes, and spinal pain and stiffness. My manipulative approach involves re-positioning the head in a more correct position relative to the rib cage, and then applying a thrust to the maximally hyperflexed upper dorsal segment.

Harrison described a move he called the "T2 drop," in which the patient lies face down on a drop-table which has the following capabilities: the cervical piece is capable of direct elevation (not simply tilting) and there is an upper dorsal droppable table section. The patient's head is first elevated on the cervical section, to a more normal position, and then a thrust is delivered to the T2 area. Although this move may appear to address the upper dorsal humping which is so apparent, and no doubt it does, at the same time it might be that the most significant effect is on the contractured anterior tissues: the anterior longitudinal ligament, the pectoral muscles, etc.

The ideal line of drive relative to the goal of stretching anterior tissues, and flattening the hump, would be more or less perpendicular to the spine. Unfortunately, such a line of drive in this region would very much approximate and compress the facets, which are very oblique to the plane line of the disk in this area of the spine. The ideal line of drive relative to the other important goal of this maneuver, mobilizing the facetal joints, would be very inferior to superior, shearing through the plane line of the facets. Unfortunately, such a line of drive would not be expected to have nearly enough of the stretching effect required for rehabilitating the contractured ALL and the other anterior tissues. In practice, when I used to use this move more, I compromised between these two conflicting criteria: at about 45^0 oblique to the spine, inferiorly to superiorly directed, balance is achieved between compressive and sheer components of the vector.

Since then, I have worked out another way of performing this maneuver, in the supine position. It does not require anything more sophisticated than a plain pelvic bench (no drop sections), a pillow, and a padded wedge, like an SOT block. The block is inserted underneath the supine patient, such that its superior aspect underlies the T2-3 interspace, or nearby, depending on that particular patient's area of maximal humping. The head most be supported, of course, by a pillow, which must be rather large for those patients that present with an unusual degree of anterior weight bearing (usually older patients). To the extent the patient can tolerate it, his or her arms are permitted to hang off the table, to the side, so that there may be some traction on the anterior tissues that need to be stretched. Indeed, it is very useful to allow the patient to lie in this position for at least a couple of minutes, so that some viscoelastic creep is achieved prior to the manipulative thrust.

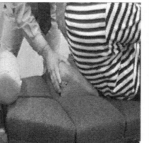 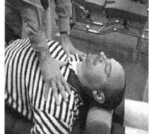

Padded wedge placement for supine AWB move.　　Anterior weight bearing move.

The doctor then takes a very broad contact with the flat of his two hands, the fingers and palms straddling the pectoral muscles, the clavicles, the sternum, as much of the anterior aspect of the shoulders as can be touched. The thrust is given very sharply, but with minimal travel distance (very much HVLA). The release which occurs is often very dramatic, equivalent to a lifetime of leaning backward against a chair, trying to crack one's own back in order to relieve the spinal tension that accompanies prolonged sitting. The doctor is advised to take it easy when using this maneuver on slender individuals, especially females, who often have more intrinsic flexibility in the costochondral joints. Less force is required, and too much force could result in an adverse consequence. The move is somewhat startling to some patients, so that very often the doctor only gets one chance to pull it off; after that, the patient is too guarded for the doctor to try again. Extra caution is also indicated to not cause female patients to feel their breast tissue is compromised; the doctor can usually arch his or her fingers above the breast tissue, or even thrust from the head of the table (although that is less effective than the more usual stance at the side of the table).

I might mention that his supine AWB move is so effective (see pre and immediate post photos), so satisfying for the patient, that it may easily seduce the doctor into forgetting all that stuff about "by hands only." In other words, this move is not meant to replace other classic means we employ to move the upper dorsal area: chair moves, diversified pisiforms, thumb moves, and all the rest. It is intended to supplement these other moves, especially when adjusting patients who come in with a significant postural abnormality, the forward head syndrome. Untreated, this problem develops into the spondylosis syndrome of later life: headaches, discogenic spondylosis, tingling in the upper extremities, and yoke pain in the shoulder girdle. Not exactly a barrel of monkeys.

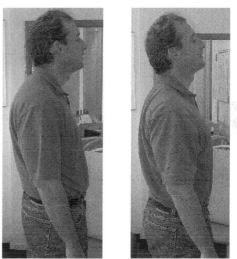

Anterior thoracic maneuver

The anterior thoracic maneuver gets increasingly more difficult to execute the higher one gets in the spine, but can be performed up to the T2 level, perhaps even T1 level. To accomplish the move this high in the spine, the doctor must lean way over the patient, aiming the thrust through the crossed arms perpendicularly to the table, right above the hand placed under the patient.

Diversified pisiform moves

The diversified pisiform move is well-known move in a general sense, but there are many variations on the same theme. Although the move is traditionally thought to correct misalignments such as those designated by PRI or PLS of T2, for me it is more about introducing a force consistent with all the examination findings. Suppose, for example, that a patient has reduced cervicothoracic lateral flexion to the right. I would put the patient prone, and then perform a local examination of the upper thoracic spine, looking for hard end-feel and/or posteriorly subluxated transverse processes. If I were to find a restricted, posterior TP on the left, I would be in the land of the modified diversified pisiform maneuver on the left. That move would introduce gross lateral flexion to the right, while simultaneously introducing movement to the fixation on the left side of the spine. If, on the other hand, I were to find a restricted, posterior TP on the *right* on this same patient, restricted in right lateral flexion, a different procedure would be required. I would have to contact the right side of the spine, while introducing a force that introduces gross lateral flexion to the right. I call the maneuvers I have worked out for this scenario a *modified* modified diversified pisiform, or modified MDP for short. Let us take a closer look at some of these moves.

At the risk of seeming excessive detailed and even confusionist, I must bring up one more qualifying factor. In the examples crafted above, there just happened to be restriction on the same side as the posterior transverse process. That simplifying assumption was made to avoid the difficult problem of what to do with criteria that point towards different strategies. What to do about a TP that is restricted, but *anterior*? I do not think a thrust on the other side of the spine would rotate the anterior TP posteriorly, nor do I think it would be efficient for introducing movement to the anterior side. I do not have any easy answers here, but simply admit I am biased in favor of emphasizing restriction as compared with misalignment. If I can not think of one adjustive procedure that could address each entity in a consistent manner, I usually go with the functional impairment, the restriction.

Modified diversified pisiform

The move introduces motion to the contacted segment, while introducing global lateral flexion to the contralateral side. The doctor assumes a so-called scissors stance alongside the cephalad end of the table, places the pisiform of the inferior hand on the ipsilateral transverse process of an upper thoracic (sometimes lower cervical) vertebra, and uses the superior hand laterally flex the patient's head and neck away from the contact hand. Notwithstanding the ritualized denunciation of scissoring – that is, using the hands in an opposed manner, so that the "stabilization hand" is actually quite involved – a *measured amount* of scissoring very much enhances the move. I do

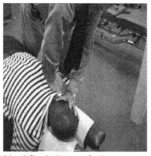

Modified diversifed pisiform.

not extend the patient's head prior to thrusting, nor do I pre-stress it very much away from my contact hand; rather, I take advantage of the fact that the patient is face down, and can not see what I am up to. Asking the patient to do anything, or applying substantial pre-stress, would eliminate the element of surprise. I keep a light touch, not much pre-stress, and then execute quickly, taking care not to press the patient's face into the head piece of the table.

Modified modified diversified pisiform

The move introduces motion to the contacted segment, while introducing global lateral flexion to the *ipsilateral* side. One possibility is to perform the traditional MDP, as described above, and simply reach across the patient to contact the opposite side of the spine. It can be done, but it is a little clumsy. It is easier to come to the head of the table, contact the posterior, fixed transverse process with one hand, the side of the patient's head with the other hand, and introduce a bilateral thrust. The doctor's elbows should be equally flexed, and the doctor should be standing at the middle of the head of the table, as compared with another style I find less effective, in which

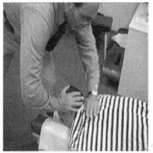

Modified modified diversified pisiform (aka head of the table move)

the doctor favors the contact side corner of the table, and essentially drags the head toward the contact hand. In doing this move as described, it is challenging to keep the contact hand on the transverse process, and avoid slipping off on to the spinous process, but one does one's best.

Diversified pisiform

This move is very similar to the MDP described above, except the contact is applied to the spinous process. I don't do this move, because the patient generally finds it uncomfortable. I have similar feelings about the thumb move, in which the doctor's thumb makes contact with the patient's spinous process. I raise no mechanical objection to either move, and congratulate those doctors who are getting the job done with them without inconveniencing the patient – I am not one of these doctors, and will not take the trouble to discuss the possible indications for these moves.

Appendix: Cervicothoracic global ROM and selecting the optimal adjustive procedure

Cervicothoracic spinal region

- Global ROM analysis
  - lateral flexion and rotation
    - ipsilateral restriction: torticollis, upper cervical rotational subluxation
    - contralateral restriction: more typical, rotary break and/or MDP
    - observe body language
- MDP and *modified* MDP
    - upper thor fix contralateral to global rest in lat bending:
      - MDP
    - upper thor fix ipsilateral to global rest in lat bending:
      - Modified MDP, from head of the table

Appendix: DD: UC vs. CT & Related adjustments

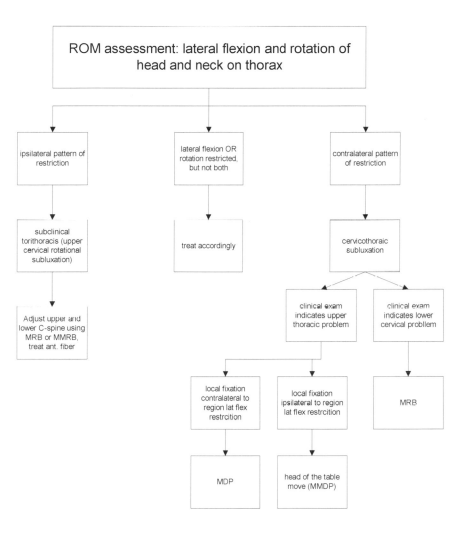

18. The cervical spine

Kinematics of the cervical spine

The upper and lower cervical spines constitutes a kinematic couple, not unlike the lumbar and thoracic spines. Their kinematic behavior is very different in the two regions, and it follows from this that there ought to be differences in our adjustive approach.

Upper cervical spine

The occipital-atlanto-axial complex includes two motor units (occ-C1, and C1-C2). Both joints participate about equally in flexion/extension, to the extent of some 10 degrees. In contrast, rotation of occ-C1 is probably less than that (Kapandji[1] says there is significant rotation, as does Grieve[2]; White and Panjabi[3] say there is none). Nonetheless, rotation at C1-C2 is large, amounting up to 50 degrees (or about half of the total for the neck). This complex in its entirety allows considerable flexion/extension (occ-C1), rotation (C1-2), and slight lateral bending (occ-C1), but also affords considerable protection of the neural elements. The IAR for rotation is very close to the spinal cord, allowing a maximum of rotation without much distortion of the cord.

When a subject rotates the neck, the motion begins from the skull and winds down the neck. Sometimes this motion restricts blood flow through the vertebral artery, which passes through the transverse process foramina, causing symptoms of cerebral ischemia (nausea, tinnitus, dizziness, vertigo, visual disturbances). In turning to the right, for example, the atlas moves anterior with respect to axis on the left, and puts a severe stretch into the vertebral artery on the left, beginning at 30 degrees. The artery is very kinked at 45 degrees. If the right side (ipsilateral, in

---

[1] Kapandji A. The Physiology of the Joints Vol 3. Edinburgh London and New York: Churchill Livingstone; 1974, p. 182.

[2] Grieve G. Common Vertebral Joint Problems. 1 ed. Edinburgh London Melbourne and New York: Churchill Livingstone; 1981, p. 43.

[3] White AA, Panjabi MM. Clinical Biomechanics of the Spine. 1st ed. Philadelphia PA: J. B. Lippincott Company; 1978, p. 66.

this case) is compromised in terms of its ability to supply blood to the brain, the occlusion of the left (contralateral) side may cause symptoms to manifest.

Lateral bending side-to-side may be as much as 8 degrees,[4] but could be considerably less than that, occurring more as linear translation of occiput on C1.[5] Lateral bending is essentially zero at C1-C2. The anterior convergence of the lateral masses and occipital condyles is what prevents rotation from occurring there, and the snug fit of the odontoid process between the anterior arch of atlas and the transverse ligament of C2 is what limits lateral flexion there. This snug fit also prevents anterior translation of C1 on C2, limiting it to 2.5 mm. in adults and 4.5 mm. in children between full flexion and extension. White and Panjabi believe that true lateral translation of C1 on C2 does not really occur, and only apparent translation, up to 4 mm., takes place during rotation at the same joint (i.e., as part of a coupling pattern).

It is generally thought that the atlas translates inferiorward on C2 during rotatory movement. This is due to the bi-convex shape of the C1-C2 articulation, in which the hyaline cartilage, if not the bony surfaces themselves, are convex on the C2 articular pillars and the lateral masses. As C1 rotates to the right, the right lateral mass drops posterior and inferior to the highest point of the C2 articulation, and the left lateral mass drops anterior and inferior to the highest point of the C2 articulation.

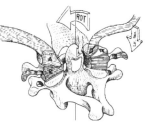

C1-2 kinematics, from Kapandji.

The coupling pattern is such that rotation and lateral bending in the upper cervical spine is *contralaterally* coupled: lateral flexion of the occiput to the right is coupled with a rotation to the left of C1 on C2. (As we shall see, this has bearing on our manipulative approach to the upper cervical area.)This is due to the fact that in rotation to the left the right atlanto-occipital ligament (which connects the inferior aspect of occiput to the anterior arch of atlas) is wrapped around the odontoid and develops tension. This tension causes in turn the flexion of the occiput to the right. Only a little rotation occurs between the occiput and C1.

Another coupling pattern which occurs is that in extension of the occiput on C1, the occiput translates anteriorly on C1, and conversely during flexion, the occiput translates posteriorly. This is due to the fact that the center of rotation for these

---

[4] White AA, Panjabi MM. Clinical Biomechanics of the Spine. 1st ed. Philadelphia PA: J. B. Lippincott Company; 1978, p. 65.

[5] Kapandji A. The Physiology of the Joints Vol 3. Edinburgh London and New York: Churchill Livingstone; 1974, p. 184.

motions is superior to the atlanto-occipital joint. (The occipital condyles are convex, sitting in the bowl-line lateral masses; the condyles slide "up the bowl" in extension, and "down the bowl" in flexion.)

Lower cervical spine

Most flexion/extension occurs in the central region, especially at C5-6, which is why this motor unit is most prone to degenerative joint disease. Motor units adjacent to those in which mobility is reduced show increased mobility and eventual degeneration. Disc degeneration in and of itself does not seem to result in loss of motion, although it may initiate a process of discogenic spondylosis in which eventual posterior joint arthrosis will limit motion. Nonetheless, all other things being equal, the taller the disc and the shorter the diameter, the greater the amount of motion that is available. In lateral flexion this diameter is measured left to right, and in flexion/extension motions, from anterior to posterior. This probably accounts at least partially for the greater mobility of the higher units of the LCS, where the disc diameters are reduced. Flexion/extension under load conditions may result in up to 2.7 mm. of linear z translation (anterior-posterior).

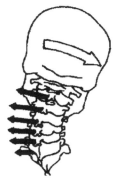

Lower cervical kinematics, from White and Panjanbi

The coupling pattern is such that the cervical bodies turn toward the side of lateral flexion, which is to say that their spinous processes turn toward the convexity of the lateral curve that is formed. (This will have implications for our manipulative approach, as did the kinematics of the upper cervical spine.) As we descend the cervical spine, there is a gradual decrease in the amount of axial rotation that accompanies any given degree of lateral bending in the opposite direction. This probably relates to the probable increasing steepness of the lower cervical facets.[6] During a bend to the right, the left inferior articular facet of the vertebra above translates anteriorly and superiorly, and the right inferior facet of the vertebra above translates posteriorly and inferiorly. This is what accounts for the ipsilateral body rotation in lateral flexion of the LCS.

The uncinate process lie in the sagittal plane, arising from the superior endplate of the vertebra at its posterior aspect, and having its articular cartilage-lined surface facing medially. They form a synovial joint with the superior lateral portions of the vertebral body of the vertebra below. The uncinate processes are thought to retard posterior translation and lateral bending excesses. Their sagittal orientation

---

[6]White AA, Panjabi MM. Clinical Biomechanics of the Spine. 1st ed. Philadelphia PA: J. B. Lippincott Company; 1978, p. 72.

is thought to "guide" anterior/posterior movement, as in flexion/extension.

In looking at the global movements of the head and cervical spine, it is necessary to make two more points. First, the manner in which a subject is able to achieve a "pure" lateral flexion is actually very complex. The LCS turns ipsilaterally, and the UCS contralaterally so that the head and eyes are able to stay in the frontal plane. Hence the UCS and the LCS are actually distinct kinematic entities (their division occurs at C2-3) that work in synchrony to perform gross balanced movements. Second, there is passive insufficiency of the sternocleidomastoid muscles which limits full flexion of the neck. This means that they are not able to elongate enough to accommodate the amount of flexion that could otherwise take place in the neck. Thus, in flexing from the shoulder region, the increasing tension on the posterior spinal ligaments and on the sternocleidomastoid muscles will eventually cause the upper cervical spine to extend. (For further amplification of these views, the reader is referred to Worth's excellent article "Movements of the Cervical Spine" in Grieve's anthology Modern *Manual Therapy of the Vertical Column*[7].)

Assessment of the cervical spine

Unlike the other spinal regions, the neck is somewhat easier to palpate with the patient supine, and so the examination methods are a little different. It is the one spinal region that we can palpate on at least three sides very easily, all but the anterior aspect readily palpable, and so we must take advantage of this opportunity for examination. The immediately following paragraphs mostly relate to assessment, but as always, the temptation to abruptly leap into adjustive procedures is irresistible, and thus somewhat indulged.

Visualization

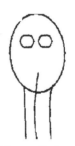

Schematic for mechanical cervicocranial inspection.

We are used to inspecting the trunk above the pelvis for the tell-tale asymmetric clefts that indicate lumbar scoliotic curvature: the side of the deeper cleft is the side of the lumbar concavity. However, we sometimes neglect to inspect the neck for precisely the same information (see right figure). If the doctor stands at the head of the table and visualizes the supine, relaxed patient, who has been straightened out as much as possible, he will often notice that one side of the neck will exhibit a certain degree of convexity, whereas the other side will be either less convex, straight, or even concave. All other things being equal, and depending on what other criteria will tell us, the

[7]Grieve G. Modern Manual Therapy of the Vertebral Column. Edinburgh London Melbourne and New York: Churchill Livingstone; 1986.

convex side will be the more optimal side to adjust, consistent with classic adjusting "on the open side of the wedge."

We see two primary cervicodorsal patterns. In the first, the upper dorsal or lower cervical spine compensates for a thoracic curvature, and itself is compensated by an opposite upper cervical curvature; the head winds up pretty much centered between the shoulders. The left figure depicts most of this.

In yet another pattern, an upper dorsal compensation for a lower dorsal curvature continues to the upper cervical area, where there is an opposite cervical curvature. The head winds up deviated toward one of the shoulders (Harrison calls this "head deviation.")This is depicted in the right figure above.

Given that the head will strike just the angle it requires on the cervical spine to level the eyes, we generally expect an "open wedge" in the upper cervical spine opposite the cervical lateral curvature of the lower cervical spine. No a priori judgement is made as to whether the cervical or thoracic lateral curvature is "primary," nor which would seem "compensatory for the other. The implications for our manipulative approach are reasonably obvious, but as always, we must temper this structural information with movement assessment, which may add impart consistent or inconsistent cues an adjusting strategy.

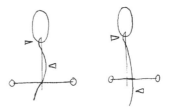

Left: cervicothoracic S-curve, head in midline
Right: cervicothoracic C-curve, with head deviation.

Motion palpation

In the case of "harder end-feel," (hypomobile motor units), the doctor notes on the side being tested a feeling akin to "the Great Wall of China." At the pain-free end point of the range of motion, there will be sudden cessation of motion and usually pain. On the more mobile side of the same or other motor units, the doctor will note a certain degree of what the motion palpators call "joint play"; that is, a rubbery pliability that may or may not cause pain on the part of the patient.

The patient is supine. The doctor places the flat of his or her hand underneath the basilar portion of the occiput, slightly elevating the head and allowing it to turn ipsilaterally. The "knife-edge" of the 2nd phalanx of the other hand is placed perpendicular to the tested side of the lower cervical spine. Care is taken to penetrate through the soft tissues so that a firm contact is made against the articular pillar.

The examiner is now in a position to test the motion characteristics of the lower cervical spine. As above, he plants one foot at the head of the table, brings the other around the corner of the table, and allows his body to smoothly glide toward the tested side. As part of the same motion, the head and neck are laterally flexed toward the tested side and contralaterally rotated. The examiner should do his best to flex laterally and rotate oppositely in one combined gesture, rather than in a jerky, two-part sequence. Should he laterally bend the neck first, rotation is relatively diminished, and vice versa.

The examiner assesses the feel at the end of the passive range of motion, and either calls which side has a harder end-feel or pronounces symmetry. The examiner is likely to note both visually and kinesthetically a difference in global coupled flexion and contralateral rotation, the lesser side corresponding to the side of harder end-feel. Once again, the doctor should not test the neck more than twice on either side, to avoid altering the presumed palpatory entity. Our own motion palpation study of the cervical spine, using continuous rather than Kappa analysis, and also using confidence calls, showed fairly good reliability using an end-feel method.

Given the accessibility of the inclinometer, one might ask why bother motion palpating at all? The obvious answer is that only manual assessment can be level-specific, at least in the absence of (invasive) stress x-rays.

Static palpation of the cervical spine

The doctor, standing at the head of the table, begins by identifying analogous left and right structures at the lateral margin of the supine patient's neck. Either the transverse processes, lamina-pedicle junctions, or articular pillars may be utilized. I prefer the transverse processes, because being the most lateral structures, there will necessarily be the greatest degree of distortion palpable. It is necessary to maneuver as much as is possible of the soft tissues out of the way, to get right on the osseous structures. The doctor decides whether the palpated structures are equally elevated off the table; he then slides up, left and right, one more unit. If the motor unit above is rotated with respect to the one above, the doctor will sense one of his palpating fingers dropping down towards the table, and the other rising up towards the ceiling. He ascends the spine using this procedure to call the vertebral rotations.

As a general rule, the upper and lower cervical spines enter into an s-shaped scoliotic pattern in a manner analogous to that of the thoracolumbar spine. We have already mentioned Worth's article in Grieve's anthology, where he contrasts the LCS from the UCS. A subluxation in the LCS will tend to be accompanied by an upper cervical subluxation on the other side of the spine. Given that hypomobile subluxations are probably more common than hypermobile subluxations, this contralateral pattern gives rise to another coarse but useful test for motion restriction. Using "pure" lateral flexion, one tests the UCS on one side simultaneously with the LCS on the other side, and then vice versa. One then decides which crossover pattern manifests the hardest end-feel, thereby evidencing the overall pattern of the neck distortion.

A few points relative to (cervical) adjusting

• It is plausible to suppose, if not actually proven, that some degree of symmetry in cervical (and spinal, in general) range of motion is preferable to significant asymmetry. We also have reason to believe[8] that lower cervical adjustments are more appropriate for ameliorating lateral bend asymmetries than upper cervical adjustments, and vice versa for rotational asymmetries. Of course, this has only been investigated using Gonstead-style chair moves, which leaves open the possibility that these site and LOD-specific effects might not carry over into another style of adjusting, such as one employing Diversified modified rotary breaks. Nevertheless, as a working hypothesis, it is suggested that the clinician approach the lower cervical spine on the side of harder end-feel.

• It is hardly an exaggeration to comment that it is not entirely clear what happens when a manipulative thrust is applied to the spine. Of course this is true in all the spinal regions, but the point seems the most telling in the cervical region, where we can literally get a *firmer grip* on the matter. Are the major articular effects on the contacted or the non-contacted side of the spine? Grieve suggests that essentially it's all in the doing. If what chiropractors' call the contact hand serves primarily as a fulcrum, then the "stabilization" hand, by accelerating the cervical structures in an opposed direction to that of the contact hand, effectuates the major articular effect: facet gapping on the "stabilized" side of the neck. If, on the other hand, the contact hand is the prime mover, with the stabilization hand remaining relatively stationary, then the major articular impact is facet shearing on the contact hand side. It would seem that anything in-between these extremes is possible, depending on the relative work performed by the two hands of the clinician. We take this into account below in describing a protocol for managing cervical intervertebral foraminal encroachment, in which the intent of the thrust is to gap the contralateral side to that of segmental contact.

• We should make another point concerning the difference between the movements of the cervical spine during voluntary motion as compared with the motion that is induced by manipulative thrusts. During voluntary rotational

[8]Nansel D, Peneff A, Quitoriano J. Effectiveness of upper versus lower cervical adjustments with respect to the amelioration of passive rotational versus lateral-flexion end-range asymmetries in otherwise asymptomatic subjects. Journal of Manipulative and Physiological Therapeutics 1992;15(2):99-105.

movement, the axis of rotation is somewhere around the spinal cord, which makes sense since we would not want to put too much stress upon it by having a pivot point too far from it. However, what happens during a manipulative thrust is most likely very different.

- The implicit and probably unjustified assumption by those performing supine (call them "Diversified") adjustments appears to be that it would be equivalent to adjust the neck from P to A on the one side, or from A to P on the other side, as though there were a central axis around which the vertebra would turn when adjusted, as in voluntary movement. Then, the audible joint releases that occur would be bilateal. However, we know that the audibles created by the modified rotatry break, and possibly other manipulative procedures, are opposite the side of contact – are unilateral.[9]

- Therefore, it is likely that when the neck is adjusted on the one side, the axis for the rotatory component is nearer to the contralateral articular pillar. Therefore, an anterior-posterior line of correction on the one side would not be equivalent to a posterior-anterior line of correction on the other side. A further implication is that the simple formulae "spinous right equals body left" and "spinous left equals body right" are probably unjustified. (We go into this at length, because it has a huge bearing on the rationale for what we describe below as the "anterior cervical break" adjustment.) In the case where the fixation is on the side of spinous rotation, it would not be appropriate to apply a massive thrust on the more mobile side in order to produce more mobility on the contralateral, fixed side. The anterior cervical move, described below, deals with the situation in which joint restriction is on the side of spinous rotation.

- The can be much patient apprehension in cervical adjusting. The head is a ten pound structure balanced on a one pound neck, with lots of small joints responsible for the overall stability for the region. The possibilities for breakdown in this region of the spine are legion, as are the possibilities for ineffective doctor interventions. The patient's unconscious neuromuscular control mechanism is fully aware of the situation. The typical patient has much greater difficulty in surrendering this area of the spine than the thoracic and lumbar spines. Very often, he is completely unable to "let it go" during examination, to the point that the head of a supine patient would remain suspended in the air if the doctor were to release it suddenly during the palpatory procedure.

- In this situation the doctor and the patient engage in a very subtle dance. When

---

[9]Brodeur R. The audible release associated with joint manipulation. Journal of Manipulative and Physiological Therapeutics 1995;18(3):155-164.

the doctor touches these structures, the patient is likely to go rigid, and were the doctor to attempt a manipulation in these circumstances, the result would almost certainly be negative. Either the adjustment would not "go," as we put it, or it would require a degree of force that is unwise. On the contrary, the doctor must back off from the patient as soon as he or she notices that the patient is guarding.

• The patient will relax, the doctor will once more make an approach, the patient will again freeze, and the doctor backs off again, and so on. These events actually take place in much less time than I am taking to describe them. The art involved is knowing how to thrust at just the right moment. A good adjustment is achieved more by obtaining minimum patient resistance than through maximal doctor intervention.

Selected cervical adjustments

I refer supine cervical manipulations to sitting and prone styles. My lower cervical repertoire consists of the conventional modified rotary break, a variation on that theme I have entitled the *modified* modified rotary break, the lateral break, and the anterior break. These moves are related to one another by being on a spectrum, that involves lines of drive that go from posterior to anterior, straight lateral to medial, to anterior to posterior. The upper cervical repertoire includes once again the modified rotary break, and two moves for the atlanto-occipital joint.

The lower cervical spine

Modified rotary break

This move is so well known that it hardly needs description, but that stated, let us say that a thrust is introduced with neck laterally flexed while the jaw is rotated toward the opposite side. In a diversified technique setting, the listing would be body left or right, and in a neo-diversified setting more concerned with movement restriction, one might say there is restriction in lateral flexion coupled with restriction in contralateral rotation. These are just the exam findings that were described above as being particularly common in the goniometric-inclinometric examination of the neck.

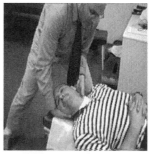

Conventional MRB, lower cervical spine.

The thrust itself may be delivered using the side of the doctor's index finger, or by turning hand around and using the thumb to pull on the articular pillar, with the other fingers more or less parallel to the jaw. I never know what to call this thumb-pull move, so I will just call it the "thumb-pull" cervical move.

The modified rotary break, using either the index finger or the thumb to introduce the force, is an *anti-synkinetic* motion (unnatural in terms of the coupling pattern) insofar as in normal kinematics the lower cervical spine couples lateral flexion to ipsilateral body rotation. Although there is no evidence that such anti-synkinesis is harmful, and allowing the possibility that such a set-up might lock up all degrees of freedom other than the one desired by the manual therapist (as the medical manipulator Carel Lewit[10] claims), I prefer set-ups that are more consistent with normal, physiologic joint motions, described below.

Modified **modified rotary break**

Although I am not aware of clinical evidence that such anti-synkinesis is harmful, I do worry about the long and short-term consequences of imposing nonphysiological movement patters on the spine. Even allowing the possibility that an asynkinetic setup locks up all degrees of freedom other than the one desired by the manual therapist (as Lewit claims), I prefer set-ups that are more consistent with normal, physiologic joint motions.

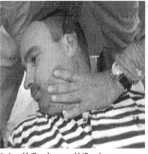

Modified modified rotary break

The modified modified rotary break (MMRB) moves the neck in a manner consistent with normal coupling patterns. The head and neck are laterally flexed away from the contacted side, and also rotated away from the contact hand. Both tissue pull and thrusting is posterior to anterior, and lateral to medial. The thumb-pull doctor's contact is easier to accomplish and better received than the index finger contact. The doctor should be at the head of the table, even though the corner is often preferred for the conventional MRB; in the MMRB, the head and neck can not be easily flexed away from the contact hand if the doctor favors the corner of the table.

Provided the doctor's fingers are positioned parallel to the jaw, the line of drive will wind up *parallel to the facets*, inferior to superior. Patients find this move particularly satisfying, in that it shears the facets so gracefully that they do not have any sense of anything having been "done to" them; the adjustment feels like it just "occurs" in some way. It is very easy to apply pre-adjustive cervical traction to the neck in this maneuver, with the fingers of the stabilization gripping the underside of the occiput and pulling away from the contact hand. It takes more rotation in the setup to take the cervical spine to tension in the MMRB compared

---

[10]Lewit K. Manipulative therapy in rehabilitation of the motor system. Washington, D.C.: Butterworths; 1985.

with the MRB.

Although I have not aware of a move like the MMRB being featured in a chiropractic technique book, field doctors tell me at continuing education seminars I teach from time to time that they deploy a procedure very similar to it. It seems that as the years of experience accumulate, many doctors come to the same conclusion I have: adjusting the necks the way they normally move feels and works better.

Which MRB to use?

Although there are precious few studies showing a difference in outcome using one manipulative procedure rather than another, it is plausible to suppose that clinical circumstances may favor certain procedures. The table lists a few factors that may bear on the optimality of either the MRB or the MMRB for the lower cervical spine.

	MRB	MMRB	comments
restriction pattern	restriction in lateral flexion and contralateral rotation	restriction in lateral flexion and ipsilateral rotation	However: the accuracy of dynamic assessment to determine fixations is very questionable (2)
high need to achieve level specificity	more preferred	less preferred	However: clinical value of segmental specificity has neen called into question (3)
high need to avoid rotation	more preferred	less preferred	less preferred
patient comfort	less preferred	more preferred	Cervical DJD especially favors MMRB
avoiding adverse consequences	less preferred	more preferred	Plausible that synkinetic manipulation is safer, especially over the long run

Notes for paragraph on MMRB

1.   Lewit K. Manipulative therapy in rehabilitation of the motor system. Washington, D.C.: Butterworths; 1985.
2.   Troyanovich SJ, Harrison DD. Motion Palpation: It's time to accept the

this that thrusting opposite the side of disc bulge may worsen the situation, presumably by causing further damage on the side of the bulge. Therefore, if the IVF encroachment we are herein discussing is thought to the consequence of disc bulge, the protocol should not be used.

Diff Di cervicobrachialgia: herniated disc vs. bony lesion

- Spurling's maneuver/cervical compression/distraction
- Neurological signs, sensory and exaggerated deep tendon reflex (if myelopathy)
- Valsava / Dejerine's triad
- X-ray (lack djd suggests herniation)
- Advanced imaging
- Bakody's sign

If, on the other hand, the IVF encroachment seems to be the result of osteophytosis, as would be confirmed by oblique cervical radiographs, then the lateral break is likely to be safe to apply to the contralateral side of the neck; even at that, prudence and restraint are recommended. Following the lateral break, I then shear the facets on the arm pain side, using the *modified* modified rotary break, with more rotation in the setup than in the thrust. There is an immediate improvement in extension, especially oblique extension toward the effected side, and often dramatic reduction in arm symptoms.

Anterior cervical move

What if the fixation in the lower cervical spine happens to be on the side of spinous process rotation? The classic Diversified strategy of applying a contact to the vertebral body on the contralateral side will not do, because what is correct from a misalignment point of view would be incorrect from a restriction point of view. The obvious solution, however unconventional the line of

---

Herman Kabat: Low Back Pain from Herniated Cervical Disc

- Occult cervical discopathy, negative myelogram and CT
- Diagnostic protocol
- Palpate thenar pads, digits 1-5 touching
- Inspect thenar pads
- Check opponens pollicis muscles, digits 1-2
- Check wrist extensors
- Check pernonius tertius
- If weakness, re-check with cervical distraction, then compression

---

drive, would be a thrust on the side of fixation, with an anterior to posterior (10% will do) component to the vector, which mostly (90%) lateral to medial.

There is yet another way of getting to this line of drive. A book by Kabat describes a syndrome akin to an occult cervical disc, in which there are standard kinesiological findings (e.g., weak wrist flexors, weak thumb opponens muscle) on the arm where there is a discopathy in the lower cervical spine. These findings are momentarily relieved by slight traction, and exacerbated by cervical compression. Kabat, writing prior to the advent of MRI, said his patients would be negative on CT scan and myelogram for discopathy. One wonders if MRI would show internal disc disruption, or what discography would show.

Having read Kabat's book, but not being particularly interested in his treatment recommendations (mostly involving avoiding certain types of movements), I looked for "his" patients, to see what listing they might have from a chiropractic point of view. I ultimately concluded that their discopathy, if indeed Kabat has got that right, involved spinous process rotation toward the side of restriction. Some practitioners of *Applied Kinesiology* have come to a similar, if not identical, conclusion, and one at least calls this "hidden cervical disk" (David Leaf). Thus, the straight mechanical indications for the anterior cervical adjustment (spinous

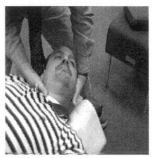
Anterior cervical break.

process = fixation) turn out to coincide with those for Kabat's hidden cervical disc syndrome. I do not know if those patients who satisfy Kabat's criteria are a subset of the SP=fixation population, if the SP=fixation patients are a subset of Kabat's criteria, or if the two populations are simply one and the same.

In the anterior cervical break, the contact point on the patient is the *anterior* aspect of the transverse process on the involved side. Although this may seem odd to some, since today's average neck is usually hypolordotic (or even partially kyphotic), and since flexion is accompanied by anterior gliding of the segment above relative to the one below, there is the obvious possibility of a segment fixating in an anteriorly subluxated position. Many chiropractors have identified such "anteriorities," at least in the cervical spine: DACBO Stonebrink, the Motion Palpation Institute, the Applied Kinesiologists, and myself.

The doctor uses an A to P tissue pull, with the head and neck flexed toward and rotated away from the contact hand, just like the setup for the conventional modified rotary break. The suggested ratio for the line of drive is 90% lateral to medial, and 10% anterior to posterior; a more dramatic A to P vector makes the adjustment too difficult to perform and is furthermore unnecessary The reader is referred to Bergmann and Zachman for discussion of a similar, but not identical, move. Students and other inexperienced adjusters are cautioned against attempting this move before having mastered the modified rotary break and the lateral break, in that order, as it is relatively difficult to perform. More conventional lower cervical adjustments may be somewhat less optimal, but will be effective enough and more comfortable for the patient until this anterior adjustment is mastered.

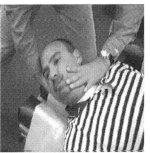

Modified rotary break, upper cervical, thumb-pull contact.

showed the examiner to be correct only 10% of the time. In view of this, if I want to adjust atlas, I roll in under the mastoid process and thrust, knowing I am doing the best I can, whether I am actually on C1 or C2.

I adjust occiput largely on *clinical grounds*, because the patient is suffering from or often suffers from tension and/or cervicogenic headaches. This would be done even in the absence of specific atlanto-occipital findings, unless there is a contraindication to a manipulative thrust at this level. That stated, I should mention that I make use of a reflex diagnostic protocol I learned from an SOT practitioner for obtaining specific atlanto-occipital listings, that modesty precludes describing in this text.

Modified rotary break (upper cervical)

For example, the primary motion that occurs in the UCS is lateral flexion coupled to contralateral rotation - therefore, the patient is pre-positioned in just this position. The set-up reproduces the physiological normal motions for the region, and there is no need to use a procedure like the *modified* modified rotary break, as described above.

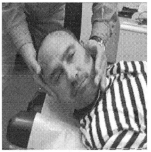

Atlanto-occipital scoop (distraction) move: the right hand is the contact, the left creates fulcrum on the mandible.

As stated above, the upper cervical spine is designed especially for rotation, coupled with contralateral lateral flexion. It would make sense to adjust it accordingly, typical atlas listings being ASRP and ASLP, unless there is good evidence that and upper cervical vertebra has subluxated in a contrary fashion. I generally adjust the upper cervical joint complex in lateral flexion and contralateral rotation. The preferred move is the thumb-pull, as described above. If, on clinical grounds, it is preferred that the LOD be either purely lateral to medial or even anterior to posterior, say for the listing ASRA or ASRP, the head is brought closer to the midline of the table or even slightly closer to the contralateral shoulder. This will lessen the degree to which the manipulative thrust effects an anti-synkinetic result.

Atlanto-occipital joint distraction move

The preferred maneuver is a lifting of the occipital condyles off the lateral mass. It may be done bilaterally, or one side if the doctor has a specific listing; I would not emphasize the significance of the headache happening to be concentrated on one side or the other. The doctor stands at the head of the table, with the patient turned *toward* the contact hand. The doctor grips the downside temporal bone by gripping the occipital area with the tips of his or her fingers and applying the palm of the hand to the temporal bone. The "stabilization" hand applies its pisiform to the angle of the patient's jaw. The thrust is delivered by a scooping movement of the occipital hand, distracting the ipsilateral atlanto-occipital joint, while the stabilization hand creates, in effect, a fulcrum at the contralateral TMJ area. Care must be taken to not accidentally manipulate the TMJ, by having the patient *clench the teeth prior to thrusting.* Scissoring is

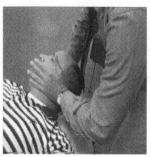

Diversified atlanto-occipital shear move.

inevitable to some extent, but that is not much of a problem; it is very difficult to train the jaw hand not to thrust at all. This is not a rotational move, and the hand on the jaw should not introduce more than minimal rotation.

Atlanto-occipital joint shear move

This is a traditional Diversified technique move, very similar to the modified rotary break applied to an upper cervical vertebra, except that the doctor applies the pisiform to the mastoid process instead.

Torticollis: differential diagnosis and treatment procedures

As a general rule, this text has not gone into specific syndromes, such as herniated disc, spondylolisthesis, nor case management very much, having elected to stick pretty much to manipulative procedures for specific segmental and regional findings. We would like to make an exception for the case of torticollis. One hears so much about spasm of the trapezius or sternocleidomastoid muscle as the cause, that one might tend to ignore the fact that what prevents the patient from flexing or turning to one side is generally *pain*, not spasm. In other words, torticollis amounts to an antalgic lean of the head and neck, and it would make no more sense to describe this as the result of spasm than it would be to ascribe the forward and laterally flexed posture of the herniated disc low back case to psoas muscle spasm.

We commented above that in torticollis, the patient is prevented from rotating or laterally flexing *toward one side.* We usually find rotational subluxation of C2-3, and have not noted any particular tendency for the vertebral body to be rotated toward or away from the side of pain, although we do not claim there is no such tendency. We simply adjust whatever we find, usually on the concave side of the cervical distortion, using a modified rotary break procedure. However, if we need to adjust on the convex side (on the side of pain), we may use the *modified* modified rotary break, even though this move is normally applied to the lower cervical spine. In this exceptional case, since the upper cervical spine cannot be flexed toward the contact hand, we contact the painful side with neck distracted away from the pain. What follows are some conditions that may emulate or result in torticollis.

Atlanto-occipital fixation

History: Head/neck trauma. Young adults common. Possibly results from a sustained awkward posture, or transitory position.

Exam findings: Head may be carried normally, or upper cervical muscle spasm might leave head in a abnormal carrying angle. Sub-occipital pain. Rotation and side flexion to the painful side are especially limited. No neurological signs, no brachial symptoms. The lateral mass may be very tender and prominent on the painful side. X-ray findings variable. The headache is confined to the suboccipital area and ipsilateral supraorbital area, whereas in fixations more caudal, the headache covers a greater area, including the entire posterior cranium on the involved side.

Treatment: Mobilization of the atlanto-occipital joint

Craniovertebral hypermobility (Grisel's syndrome)

History: "Wry-neck" might be first sign of juvenile RA. Inflammation involving the atlas transverse ligament allows anterior hypermobility of atlas on axis. Same clinical presentation may occur in URI, tonsilitis, pharyngitis, which produce same weakening of the transverse ligament (Grisel).

Exam findings: X-ray diagnostic. May be increase in retropharyngeal space from 6 to 20 mm. Cervical lymphadenopathy. HA.

Treatment: Movement treatments are contraindicated. Treatment must be directed toward the underlying pathology.

Adult RA (neck involvement)

History: RA demonstrates 40% neck involvement. Atlas-axis involvement reported at 25%.

Exam findings: X-ray shows >3mm separation of anterior tubercle and odontoid on flexion film. Perhaps 20% show platybasia (tip of dens more than 4.5mm superior to McGregors line, which is drawn from posterior edge of hard palate to most inferior aspect of occiput). Suboccipital pain with radiation to other cranial areas. Neurologic signs may result from vertebral artery occlusion, or compressive effects of RA lesions on nerves. These may include vertigo, facial sensory loss, arm/leg paresthesia, difficulty walking, urgency in micturition, and TIAs.

Treatment: Surgery, rigid cervical collar. Very cautious manual therapy if radiological stability demonstrated.

Rotational subluxation of C1/C2.

History: Trauma common cause. Awkward motions or abnormal sleep postures may provoke the condition. It may also follow URIs (Grisel's syndrome). There is occipital and hemicranial pain, facial pain/paresthesia, HA.

Exam findings: "Outstanding radiological feature is that of fixation of the *atlas* on the axis in a relationship normally attained to a greater or lesser degree during rotation ... Fixation in a position possible to a normal neck." (Grieve, CVJP, p.212). "Atlantoaxial rotatory displacement is a common cause of torticollis in childhood, and almost all patients recover spontaneously from the condition even without treatment" (Fielding, J Bone & Joint Surg, 58A:400, 1976). Head and neck may be normally aligned, especially if the condition is chronic. X-ray would show C1/C2 rotational subluxation. Painless hard end-feel may be detected. Some patients may have postural tilt to one side and rotation to the other (i.e., the normal kinematic posture for upper cervical coupled lateral flexion and contralateral rotation). These may have the *contralateral* SCM (which is stretched) in a hypertonic but futile effort at counteracting the altered posture. This distinguishes it very clearly from spasmodic torticollis in which the *ipsilateral* SCM is the deforming force.

Treatment: Manual therapy should be gentle at first, and leads to cautious mobilization of the C1-C2 joint.

Acute torticollis or wry-neck

History: Usually C2-3, but may be a more inferior motor unit. May be arm involvement. Pain radiates into shoulder area from upper cervical area as day develops. May follow prolonged stretching, as in an abnormal sleep posture. Onset very variable, from minor trauma, upon waking, sleeping in front of an open window, etc. Patient may report hearing a "click" at onset of problem. Theories for mechanism include meniscoid block, local irritability without a meniscoid block, and disc bulging resulting from viscoelastic creeping. (cf.

Cyriax). Type 1 is of sudden onset (probably a meniscoid block), and type 2 is noted on waking in the morning (probably a disc lesion).

Exam findings: Antalgic lean away from side of pain, with some anterior flexion as well. Ipsilateral arm elevation may be painful or restricted. Neck is slightly flexed and rotated away from the side of pain, a little flexed. The pain in type 1 is unilateral at pillar on neck, no radiation to arm or neck yoke area. Pain in type 2 does spread to these

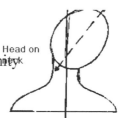

Upper cervical wry neck

areas. The "head on neck" deformity indicates an upper cervical lesion, whereas the "neck on thorax" posture indicates a lower cervical lesion. There may be rotation away from the lesioned side. "The phenomenon of blocking tends to prevent the joint closing down, or approximating the joint surfaces but does not

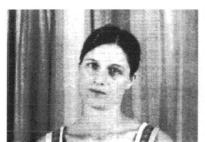

From McNair, in Grieve's MMT, p.34.

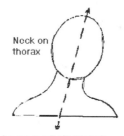

Lower cervical wry neck

Upper vs. lower cervical torticollis

apply to opening up the joint or distracting the surfaces" (McNair, in Grieve's MMT, p.354).

Treatment: Localized mobilization. Some patients benefit from a soft support. Manipulative thrusts are safe if the symptoms are minor, the exact segment has been ascertained, and there is no history of significant trauma. Usually applied to *concave* side of deformity (non-painful side). Type 1 may be relieved in a single manipulation, whereas type 2 may be more protracted, and require traction at some point. For type 1, the head and neck may be pulled toward the side of less pain. The structures are brought toward the neutral position as the pain and spasm subside. Cervical rotation is initially effected away from the side of pain.

Spasmodic torticollis

History: Rare.

Exam findings:
SCM 75% of cases, trapezius 50%. Other muscles may include RCPM, inferior capitis, and splenius capitis.

Treatment: whatever works, including medical referral for pharmaceutical approach with muscle relaxants.

19. The Temporomandibular Joint

Although there are some scholarly descriptions available on the functional anatomy of the temperomandibular joint (TMJ) , they do not tend not easily lend themselves toward treatment options. Fortunately a relatively few guiding principles will guide the clinician toward a safe and effective means of addressing this joint. For some reason, some clinicians do not like addressing this joint manually, and reach for their adjusting instruments when they feel something needs to be done. In my view, this is not necessary.

Many TMJ problems are related to slippage of the articular disc which normally remains between the condyle of the jaw and the glenoid fossa of the skull.

History

The patient may complain of bilateral or unilateral jaw pain, ringing in the ears (tinnitus), fatigue on chewing or talking, headache, popping noises during jaw movements, and other varied symptoms. The onset is usually gradual, but may be related to a trauma. There is a clinical entity called mandibular whiplash, generally associated with motor vehicle accidents. It is not uncommon for the patient to report a history of recent dental work. That may seem to have gone forward without complications, but within a day or two TMJ symptoms may set in.

```
TMJ evaluation and treatment

History:
        Jaw pain, fatigue on chewing/talking,
        tinnitus, popping, headache, difficulty closing
Inspection
        Mandible deviation (static)
        Mandible deviation opening/closing
Palpation (anterior to or in ear)
        Pain/tenderness
        Opening/closing rhythm
Treatment
        Myofascial tx, Muscles of mastication
        Manipulations: Supine thrust for PS-jaw,
        sitting lift for AI-jaw
```

Inspection

The jaw should be inspected from a few feet away by means of the doctor directly gazing at the patient, who holds the jaw relaxed but closed. The position of the midpoint of the mandible is assessed in relation to another cranial landmark, generally the nose; so long as the inspector is aware that the nose itself is often deviated. Sometimes one can do no better than to judge the position of the jaw in relation to the entire cranium, best as one can. A positive finding would mean the jaw is deviated to one side or the other.

After assessing the static position of the jaw, the doctor should next carefully observe the process of jaw opening. The patient is asked to slowly open the jaw while the doctor looks for evidence of deviation on opening toward one side or the other. Both simple and complex pathways can often be visualized as the jaw opens fully, ranging from a C curve to an S curve to even more complicated pathways. I am most concerned with how the jaw behaves at the initiation of opening, and less concerned with the pathway it takes upon being fully opened. The return pathway during jaw closing is generally the opposite of that seen during opening, but this need not necessarily be the case.

It almost goes without saying, but it is worth pointing out that the doctor should be on the lookout for visible signs of trauma and inflammation, which when present may reflect infection. I did have a case one time of a patient self-presenting with a putative TMJ problem, actually thought to be so by her dentist, whom I ultimately determined to have a abscess near the site of recent dental work. I sent her in to an emergency dental clinic for immediate administration of antibiotics, and continue to be puzzled as to why her dentist would have recommended seeing a chiropractor for a "TMJ problem."

Palpation

In addition to generic soft-tissue palpation around the jaw joints, looking for signs of inflammation and swelling, it is important to assess the mandibular gait, the process of jaw opening and closing. As a general rule, the impression of the mandibular gait ascertained during inspection will be corroborated through palpating opening and closing. This is easily done with the doctor standing behind the patient, with fingers bilaterally placed on the mandible just anterior to the mastoid processes. The jaw can also be easily felt by means of fingers placed inside the external auditory canal, but this is less preferred, in that patients do not like the feeling very much, nor is it entirely sanitary without precautions.

Diagnosis (listings)

From a static analysis point of view, the jaw is diagnosed as being either anterior-inferior (AI) on the one side or postero-superior (PS) on the other. The AI jaw is related to posterior subluxation of the disc, resulting in difficulty closing the teeth tightly. The PS jaw is related to anterior subluxation of the disc, and results in opening hesitation and clicking. As is typically the case in clinical chiropractic, the doctor simply feels an asymmetry in the static or dynamic performance of the left and right joints; which side is judged to be of clinical interest, is determined in a word to be the "listing," is related to the side and severity of symptoms. From that point of view, the history if very important. Observing an AI/PS listings couple, the side to be addressed, or at least emphasized in treatment, will be the side of greater symptoms: pain, tinnitus, fatigue, etc.

The side of initial opening, which almost always corresponds to the side contralateral to mandibular deviation, is an AI jaw, whereas the side of delayed opening, which is the side to which the jaw deviates on opening, is the PS jaw. Treatment vectors are determined by this judgement.

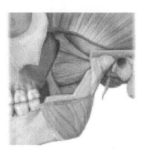

Muscles of mastication: masseter, temporalis, medial pterygoid, and lateral pterygoid

In addition to the static and dynamic findings, the doctor should carefully palpate the muscles of mastication for tender and trigger points. There is invariably a myofascial aspect to TMJ dysfunction, to the point that treating the muscles may be the only treatment required. The internal pterygoid is hard to access, but the others present no such problems.

It is my impression that the PS jaw is more likely to be primary than the AI jaw, if for no other reason than people tend to carry a lot of "nervous tension," an interesting phrase, in their muscles of mastication. That is, hypertonic jaw closing muscles often related to stress and resultant anxiety and anger result in a fixated, PS jaw. I usually find the AI diagnosis more related to mechanical trauma, and less common.

Treatment

There are manipulative procedures described for each of the listings. The AI jaw is corrected either supine or with the patient seated, by means of the doctor thrusting toward the jaw joint using hands cupped under the mandible. The patient is asked to slowly close the jaw, and the doctor executes a short thrust at about midpoint of jaw closure. The PS jaw is corrected supine, by means of an HVLA thrust (relatively gentle) executed by the doctor's pisiform on the angle of the jaw. The mechanical vector for the thrust is pretty much identical to that which is used in the modified rotary break; the main difference is that the hand is turned around so that the pisiform, rather than the side of the index finger, makes contact with the angle of the jaw.

In addition to the thrusting procedure, it is very helpful to use resisted stretching to relax the muscles of mastication, specifically on the side of a PS jaw. I cup the chin with both hands, not unlike the setup for adjusting the AI jaw, and then apply a sustain pull inferiorly and away from the side of the PS jaw, instructing the patient to resist with perhaps 20% of their possible force. This is simply a variety of proprioceptive neurofacilitation (PNF). It is not particularly necessary to determine which of the muscles is the primary offender, since whichever of them is offending is going to be treated in this manner.

Finally, it will also be helpful to use digital pressure to identify tender points in the muscles, as visualized in the anatomical drawing above. Ischemic pressure and goading in various directions will reduce the level of myofascial dysfunction in the muscles of mastication, and other muscles of facial expression that may play a role in the overall situation. The doctor will have to don a finger cot if he or she intends to work on any of internal pterygoid muscle, inside the oral cavity. The patient can be given instructions to work at massaging and stretching their own muscles at home.

Appendix 1. Chiropractic radiology

Analytic and diagnostic x-rays

X-rays have always been controversial and divisive in chiropractic, ever since Loban led a number of students to literally secede from the Palmer College in the early years, out of opposition to the introduction of x-ray into the practice of chiropractic (the protesters must have thought x-ray was a medical procedure). There are certain indications for taking diagnostic x-rays upon which all chiropractors would agree: ruling out fractures, infections, tumors, etc.

X-rays not only help render the differential diagnosis, but rule out contraindications to manipulation and other forms of chiropractic treatment. Where it gets sticky is whether analytic x-rays should be taken for the purpose of obtaining listings. Studies have shown x-rays to correlate very poorly with pain and other patient complaints. Furthermore, there is scant evidence that improvements in patients' symptoms track changes in their x-rays. there is no evidence that the outcome of care is made better by the practice of taking x-rays to establish listings, whereas there are some good reasons to consider exposure to ionizing radiation a biohazard. Although some believe analytic x-rays to represent an unnecessary expense more likely to turn up red herrings than valuable clinical information, others remain dumbfounded as to how a chiropractor could profess to do well without them.

There are two primary questions raised that continue to instigate heated discussion: first, does the safe and effective practice of chiropractic require x-rays for biomechanical analysis; and second, what is the likelihood that routine radiographs, not taken in relation to red flags being present, will exhibit previously unsuspected and important pathology?

Analytic roentgenometrics: friend or foe?

Although many investigators have questioned the traditional methods of chiropractic x-ray marking, it remains a very common practice among doctors and chiropractic interns to use such methods to generate chiropractic listings. These listings, of course, wind up dictating the lines of drive that are employed in chiropractic adjustments. Although most clinicians employ a variety of diagnostic procedures in addition to spinography, it would be hard to exaggerate the importance of the latter in determining which segments are adjusted and in which direction. This remains true in spite of the fact that many investigators have found only the most tenuous connection between x-ray findings and spinal dysfunction. Moreover, others have called into question the importance of "misalignment" as a criterion for a chiropractic adjustment, and a spinographic protocol that would be based upon it. Additional arguments against the routine use of x-ray to generate listings are based upon the prevalence of anatomic asymmetry, patient positioning errors, non-alignment of x-ray equipment, and the difficulty of achieving acceptable interexaminer reliability in the marking of the films.

This plethora of doubt concerning the value of analytic roentgenometrics has led many within the profession to advocate abandoning such methods altogether. However, it would be more prudent to judge each of the various spinographic interpretive procedures on its own merits rather than rush to judgement on the value of the process per se. Although roentgenometric findings may be a poor predictor for spinal dysfunction, this does not rule out the possibility that taking their implications into account when electing for a particular segmental contact and line of drive may evoke a more satisfactory clinical outcome than not doing so. One thing is certain: in order to generate testable hypotheses concerning the value of x-ray marking procedures, clinicians will first have to erect a body of gold standards.

X-ray reliability and validity issues

Although it is common to find the reliability of x-ray line marking called into question, that, in our opinion, is not the problem; we are persuaded that patients can be positioned in a reproducible manner, and that x-ray line-markers can find agreement on the distances and angles on the films. No doubt there are differences in the reproducibility of the various x-ray and line marking protocols, but we are satisfied that most of the problems are soluble on that level.[1] The primary problem with chiropractic analytic radiology has to do with its validity: whether the various measurements accurately describe the flesh and blood patient, and whether the use of x-rays improves the outcome of care. In other words, as an example, although doctors may agree that one innominate bone is indeed taller than the other, have we adequately demonstrated that such a longer innominate bone on x-ray identifies a posterior rotation of the innominate bone, as Gonstead and other doctors believe? (See appendix 2.)

---

[1] Harrison DE, Harrison DD, Troyanovich SJ. Reliability of spinal displacement analysis of plain X-rays: a review of commonly accepted facts and fallacies with implications for chiropractic education and technique [see comments]. J Manipulative Physiol Ther 1998;21(4):252-66.

There have been very few studies on the how valid the x-ray line marking rules are, and none to our knowledge confirming the clinical value of analytic x-rays. (Again, appendix 2 describes my own study of one of the more cherished line marking rules.) Lacking data, in the short term, we will have to use our common sense to determine whether particular line marking rules are reasonable or not. For example, there is good reason to believe that IN and EX markings for the innominate bone would be exquisitely sensitive to Y axis rotation, as one sacroiliac joint becomes more sagittally oriented than the other more coronally oriented joint. On the other hand, it is hard to imagine how Y axis rotation would produce the artificial impression of a lateral flexion malposition (i.e., open wedge), when such a malposition occurs in isolation from the more normally aligned joints above and below.

Patient positioning

It is far from obvious, in interpreting x-rays analytically, how one might distinguish asymmetry on the film due to positioning artifact as compared with patient subluxation. Special x-ray setups and computer-assisted radiometric techniques have been developed, but these are expensive, error prone in themselves, and beyond the reach of the average chiropractor. We have not been impressed with the various rules that have been put forward that supposedly help us establish that the patient was positioned well, so that any visible radiographic asymmetry reflects patient subluxation. Such rules include looking at the greater trochanters, seeing if the sacral apex bisects the symphysis, looking at the lateral skull borders, etc.

Indeed, we find ourselves frequently examining the patient carefully in order to interpret the films, a complete inversion of the more typical procedure of taking radiographs to interpret the patient. This is to some extent the approach of Hildebrandt in his excellent text Chiropractic Spinography[2], and the reason we admire it so much. We must directly confront the problem that there is an irreducible and inevitable fallacy implicit within the methodology of arbitrarily selecting any unit of the spine, defining it as an origin, and determining misalignment values of other units of the spine with respect to this origin. Let us give an example.

"Careful" x-ray positioning: a case in point

We provide an upper cervical example of the implicit problem in x-ray interpretation. Assume an individual with one misalignment: atlas is rotated

---

[2]Hildebrandt RW. Chiropractic Spinography. 2nd ed. Baltimore: Williams & Wilkins; 1985.

spinous left (aka body right) with respect to axis, and the skull sits on top of atlas without a problem. This person therefore presents with head rotation to the right. Let this patient wander into an upper cervically oriented office; let him be put in a chair, have his head clamped, and the chair rotated to the left until the ears are evenly visible from the x-ray tube; now, take the film. When the film is analyzed, one will note that atlas and occiput are "zeroed" (i.e., non-misaligned); however, there is a left rotatory cervical scoliosis, due to the fact that the normal lordosis has been positioned pointed left with respect to the x-ray tube. This person may receive a body left adjustment to the mid-cervical spine; likewise, in an upper cervical x-ray analysis, he will be said to present with a "lower angle." Since by our assumption the only misalignment present in this patient is an atlas rotated spinous left, this mid-cervical "misalignment" is an artifact of this doctor's devotion to aligning the cranium to the x-ray tube.

Let this same patient wander into another office where he is positioned by having him back up until some part of his body - the buttocks, thoracic spine, or shoulders - touches the cassette. Will not the neck now project as normal, with the atlas and cranium rotated to the right, and therefore subluxated? By our initial assumption, which is that the only misalignment is that atlas is rotated spinous left, this doctor is correct.

Now let a third doctor, lacking the assumed information that atlas is rotated spinous left, be asked to review these two sets of films. It turns out that he has no way of distinguishing a normal atlas with a left rotatory cervical scoliosis, from an atlas rotated spinous left with an otherwise straight cervical spine. He would have to visualize the patient, to see if the neck had an obvious convexity, or if the head were rotated with respect to an otherwise bilaterally symmetric body. In short, the third doctor needs to visualize the patient to interpret the x-rays.

Let us now imagine that another patient walks into the upper cervical office, this time presenting with a left convex rotatory curvature in the cervical spine, with an atlas-occiput complex that is not misaligned with respect to

The paradox of x-ray positioning: how to distinguish accurate radiograph of subluxated patient from inaccurate radiograph of normal patient, and anything in-between.

the odontoid, nor presenting with any other misalignments. The doctor puts the patient in the chair, and discovers that he does not need to rotate the chair to take the film. What does the film look like? Amazingly enough, it is identical to the image of the first patient, the one with right head rotation and no other misalignments: left rotatory convexity of the neck, normal atlanto-occipital alignment! We might even imagine a third patient, presenting with a left convex rotatory curve, and a left rotated head on atlas: he is placed in the chair, rotated to the right, and lo and behold, his x-ray shows no misalignment!

If, as in our example of the first doctor, we align a subluxated segment or region of the spine to the x-ray tube, than other areas of the spine will appear to be subluxated which in fact may not be. Or, if we "align" the non-subluxated areas of the spine to the tube, even if by accident, as in the case of our second doctor, then the true misalignment may be characterizable from the film.

In the example at hand, the upper cervical office, which positions its patients by aligning the skull to the central ray of the x-ray tube, by turning the seated patient on a chair, finds Patients 1 and 2 to share identical spinal configurations, even though they are truly different. The upper cervical office furthermore concludes that Patient 3, with deviations of both the upper cervical spine and the lower cervical spine, to have a normal cervical spinal configuration. The less rigorous Diversified office, which radiographs patients "as they usually stand," produces radiographs which are more suggestive of the patients' actual spinal configurations.

Risk-benefit analysis for x-ray

One would have to be a specialist in the field to form an independent opinion as to the true biohazard represented by x-rays. The pendulum seems to swing back and forth, from decade to decade, from x-ray posing a significant health threat to x-rays being quite safe. For anyone who is not a specialist in the field, anyone who has not had the opportunity to pore through what primary research there is on the health hazards, the expert opinions of those who have had this opportunity will just have to do. Unfortunately, the "experts" tend to look at the same data and come to diametrically opposed conclusions, just as do on the vaccination issue, which is perhaps even more emotionally explosive among chiropractors than the x-ray issue.

In the meantime, it would certainly be prudent to not take more x-rays than are necessary, and to use an x-ray technique that minimizes the patient exposure. I do not take any x-rays for the purposes of obtaining listings (again, identifying pathology, from cancer to IVF encroachment, is a different matter), having come to the conclusion that there is more than enough information available from other examination methods to know what to do from a clinical point of view. On the other hand, if a patient walks in with x-rays taken elsewhere, for whatever reason, I will certainly go over them carefully for evidence of misalignment, etc. My sense of being able to dispense with analytic x-rays is partially the result of having satisfied myself, by comparing x-rays with flesh and blood patients, that physical examination methods, tempered by knowledge of anatomy and an appreciation of coherent spinal distortion patterns, adequately predict x-ray findings. That is a testable hypothesis, not to our knowledge tested as of yet, with the somewhat relevant exception of McKenzie examination methods predicting discograms.

Appendix 2. Actual and projected innominate length

Chiropractic radiometrics: a case in point

Right from the beginning chiropractors insisted that the concept of subluxation, whatever other characteristics it may have, absolutely must embody the idea of misalignment. Not surprisingly, they expected that the radiograph to represent their gold standard; the federal government came to the same conclusion by 1974, when it included chiropractic within Medicare on the condition that the claimant be able to show the government the subluxation - the bone out of place - on x-ray.

Even the staunchest of advocates of subluxation *qua bone-out-of-place* would have to admit that the roentgenometric backup has been elusive, at best. There is very little evidence, at least to date, that adjustments reposition bones. Perhaps this explains the drive toward reliability studies that would show that chiropractors can agree on x-ray marking: since we can't seem to demonstrate that the bones move, maybe we can at least agree on *where* they are. After interexaminer reliability in x-ray marking is established, we'll try to figure out why we needed to mark the x-rays so carefully in the first place. Reliability first, then on to validity, right?

I have not been comfortable with the idea of developing measuring tools independently of their anticipated utility. That's a little like devoting your whole life preparing for the *return* of extra-terrestrials. Who cares if chiropractors can agree on their x-ray marking, unless there's *a priori* reason to believe that positional alterations of known magnitude, consistent with physiological joint motions, would indeed produce measurable roentgenometric displacements? When it comes to developing chirometric (measuring) technology, necessity should be the mother of invention. That's why I worked out a kinesiological hypothesis for the Derifield pelvic leg check (see chapter above), knowing full well I was trying to explain a phenomenon not fully shown to exist. There would be no reason to work out a reliable Derifield leg check, unless there was a plausible, physiological model indicating that such a check could in principle yield important clinical information.

Frustrated by the fact that there was continuous chatter about whether x-ray line marking was reliable, but virtually no discussion of the inherent reasonablity of what the x-ray marking systems were supposed to indicate about the patients, I decided to check out the validity of at least one well-known golden goody of x-ray marking, as a case in point: the rule that a posteriorly-rotated innominate would project with a relatively greater vertical length on the AP radiograph. More precisely, I set out to disprove this rule, which I believed to be an artifact of an anatomical mistake that went back to

Logan. My partial failure to do so was in itself a successful bridge to some really interesting and clinically valuable information.

A cherished x-ray line marking rule, reconsidered

The purpose of the present study was to scrutinize one of the better-known x-ray marking conventions, a representative statement of which is as follows: "When an ilium misaligns in a PI direction, the length of the innominate involved increases on the A-P film" (1).

The idea behind this rule is likely attributable to Logan.(2) He found that assuming an original inferior-anterior subluxation of the sacrum, that the innominate bone would eventually experience an "eccentric rotation" posteriorly (3). This conception is an obvious predecessor to the more current nomenclature "PI ilium," an expression that Logan himself never used. He went on to state that "holding the sacrum and innominate in the position they normally assume in the body," and furthermore assuming an axis for pelvic torsion "at some point between the acetabulum and the center of the sacro-iliac articulation," that a line drawn from this axis to the highest point of the iliac crest would run anterosuperiorly. This would mean that a posterior rotation of the innominate bone would raise the

Figure 1. Iliac crest height as function of location of axis of innominate rotation. Crest elevates in Logan model (left), but moves inferiorward in Hildebrandt model (right).

crest of the ilium on the involved sign (Figures 1,2). Logan apparently believed that if the greatest innominate length became more vertically oriented, then the x-ray projection would have to reflect this fact by itself as well measuring longer. He did not realize that this would not always be true, that it depended on how the patient was positioned relative to the central ray (as we shall see below).

Logan's belief that the posteriorly rotated innominate would display a greater vertical measurement on x-ray (4) carried over into the work of Gonstead (5). The latter had the sacroiliac joint constituting the axis of rotation for pelvic torsion, and the longest dimension of the innominate bone in the sagittal plane view running anterosuperiorly from the ischial tuberosity to the iliac crest. Under these assumptions, the vertical length of the innominate would have to increase given a posterior-inferior rotation of the PSIS (Figure 1).

Figure 2. Logan's gaff.

Gonstead did not to my knowledge specify any normal carrying angle of the pelvis, as did Logan, in spite of the fact that this turns out to have a critical bearing on the roentgenometric assessment of pelvic torsion.

The fact that something is amiss in the Logan-Gonstead formulation is made evident if we compare Logan's drawing of the basic postural distortion (Figure 4) with that of almost any other worker, say, that of Kendall and McCreary (6) (Figure 3). One notices how exceeding awkward it is to draw the innominate bone elevated ipsilateral to the inferior sacrum, as did Logan. It also seems rather dysfunctional to have the lumbar spine incline toward the side of the elevated iliac crest. Kendall's drawing, on the other hand, corresponds to a well-behaved Lovett-positive. According to Erhardt, "Lovett positive is the least offending and is a normal compensatory deviation" (7).

Figure 3. From Kendal and McCreary.

The most cogent account of the roentgenometric projection characteristics of the PI ilium has been produced by Hildebrandt (8). His point of departure is an original, anatomically correct description of the mechanics of pelvic torsion, in which the axis of rotation transects the symphysis pubis. He shows that if this axis were posteriorly located, say near the hip or SI joint as in the Logan-Gonstead formulation, the symphysis pubis would exhibit a sheering of which it is generally incapable (Figure 4). Although his drawing credits Gonstead with an acetabular pivot, the extreme stress upon the interpubic ligaments would be even more pronounced for the sacroiliac axis claimed by Herbst (representing the Gonstead conception).

In Hildebrandt's alternative description of pelvic torsion, the iliac crest is lowered on the side of the inferior sacrum, opposite from Logan but consistent with virtually all contemporaneous descriptions such as that of Kendall and McCreary. It is interesting to note that as the innominate rotates posteriorly, all points within it move inferiorward. The symphysis is spared.

Changes in *actual* innominate vertical length

Against this backdrop of historical information it was decided to geometrically calculate innominate height changes as a function of pelvic torsion. Hildebrandt's pelvic torsion model, in which the paired innominate bones "cleave" about a symphysis pubis axis, was selected for the analytic engine. Furthermore, it was necessary to formulate a hypothesis as to the normal carrying angle of the pelvis and sacrum, because innominate height changes turn out to be a function not only of the degree of pelvic cleavage but also of the pelvic/sacral carrying angle. For the purposes of this study it does not matter whether we use as a reference point the degree of bilateral pelvic tilt (as a unit) or the plane line of the sacral base in the sagittal view, either serving as surrogate for the other.

Figure 4. The analytical engine is based on Kapandji's drawing of the innominate bone.

The variables are defined as follows:
A = nml innom. angle, with ASIS=PSIS
B = nml ischial angle, with ASIS=PSIS
C = innom sub. angle (shown as PI)
H_{ci} = initial crest height
H_{ct} = torsional crest height
H_c = dec. crest height, post-torsion
H_{Ii} = initial ischial height
H_{It} = height ischium, post-torsion
H_I = dec. ischial height, post-torsion
R_c = radius of the crest
R_i = radius of the ischium

Some authorities believe that normally speaking the pelvis is carried such that the ASISs and the PSISs are carried at the same height, left and right (12,13). Others (14, 21), would have the ASIS and the symphysis pubis in the same vertical line, in order that the pull of the rectus abdominis and rectus femoris muscles be parallel. After examining several published drawings of sagittal views of innominate bones, it was determined that

Kapandji's drawing of the medial aspect of the innominate bone best satisfied both criteria: the ASIS and pubis were lined up, as were the ASIS and PSIS (15). Accordingly, this drawing was selected as a basis for the computations. Simple trigonometry was used to calculate innominate length changes:

$$\text{(innom length)} = Hc - Hi = Rc \{\cos A - \cos(A+C)\} - Ri \{\sin B - \sin(B+C)\}$$

Computations were performed for 3 bilateral pelvic tilt angles (pelvic carrying angles):

0^0 = normal pelvic carrying angle, PSIS = ASIS and ASIS = pubis
-10^0 = anterior bilateral pelvic tilt ("steep")
$+10^0$ = posterior bilateral pelvic tilt ("flat").

It should be noted that the values that are calculated are for actual innominate height changes, not x-ray projected changes. These values can be read off the graphs in Figure 6, (which also show the data for x-ray projections). It can be seen that the innominate length changes with posterior rotation are not impressive, except perhaps in the case of large subluxations in a steep-angled pelvis. Furthermore, sometimes the innominate vertical length decreases as the bone rotates posteriorly (flat pelvic carrying angles). It would take further calculations to determine how x-ray projections of these innominate rotations bear on the interpretation of the results.

More impressive numbers would result if one assumed opposed, bilateral rotations of the innominate bones; that is, one rotates PI while the other simultaneously rotates AS. There is a study by Cibulka et al in which this sort of intrapelvic distortion was measured (13), but some methodological problems make the study hard to interpret.

Changes in *projected* innominate vertical length

This phase enlarges upon the previous one by focusing upon the roentgenometric data; that is, it computes projected innominate length changes, which turn out to be very sensitive not only to the PCA, but also to the FFD and direction of the central ray.

The projected vertical length of the innominate bone turns out to be a function of three initial conditions: (1) the location of the x-ray tube, in terms of FFD and direction of the central ray (CR); (2) the amount of intrapelvic innominate torsion (roughly, "AS/PI" innominate subluxation); and (3) the pelvic carrying angle (PCA) of the subject (bilateral anterior or posterior pelvic tilt). (Assume no Y axis rotation.)

• A "normal" PCA is defined as one in which the ASISs and the PSISs are level, and/or the symphysis pubis and the ASISs are on the same vertical line. "Steep" and "flat" PCAs are defined as 10^0 bilateral pelvic tilt anteriorly or posteriorly.

• The symphysis pubis is defined as the origin of a Cartesian coordinate system in which the position of the following landmarks, taken from a drawing by Kapandji, are givens and expressed as pairs of coordinates: the maximum height of the iliac crest (crest peak), the minimum height of the ischium (ischial base), and the PSIS.

A spreadsheet is used to calculate the projected length of the innominate bone as different values are assigned to the location of the x-ray tube, the degree of intrapelvic torsion, and the PCA of the subject. The overall system is dynamic, in the sense that the horizontal position of both the film and the x-ray tube shift as the innominate bone rotates in the (more or less) sagittal plane, this in order to maintain a constant FFD and keep the film pressed against the PSIS even as the innominate moves. Furthermore, the vertical position of the tube also changes to maintain itself either one inch below the iliac crest (sectional radiographs) or in a defined relationship to the innominate dimensions (APFS radiographs). If CPs and IBs refer to the peak of the subluxated ilium and the base of the subluxated ischium, respectively, then the elevation of the CR above the symphysis pubis is given by the following formula: CRy = 1.5(CPs - IBs).

The sagittal plane projectional aspects of pelvic cleavage are shown in Figure 5, and some of the data are shown in Table 1. Positive values on the x axis represent degrees of unilateral posterior innominate rotation. Positive values on the Y axis represent millimeters of projected innominate length increases (the actual innominate is standardized at 200 mm).

It may be observed that:

• projected innominate length is a monontonically increasing function of posterior innominate rotation for normal and steep PCAs. Full-spine radiography produces magnitudes about double that of sectional

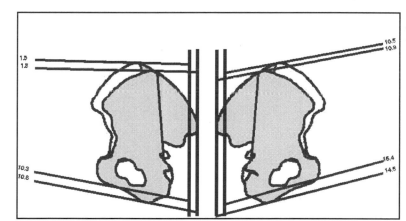

Figure 5. In both the AP lumbopelvic and the APFS pelvic projections, the vertical length of the innominate bone increases as it rotates posteriorly about a symphysis pubis axis. The relative increase is greater in the case of the APFS projection, largely because the innominate bone is more off the central ray. This effect would have been more extreme had a bilaterally anteriorly tipped pelvis been depicted, and less apparent - or even *reversed* - had a bilaterally posteriorly tipped pelvis been illustrated. The degree of innominate torsion also exerts an influence. The numbers above are normalized for a standard 200 mm innominate vertical length. Although a rather massive posterior subluxation is shown for the sake of clarity, the x-ray beam angles are drawn quite accurately for the respective projections.

radiography for any given degree of subluxation.

• For a flat PCA, full-spine radiography shows a slightly increasing innominate length. Interestingly, this is true in spite of the fact that actual innominate vertical length decreases in such an individual as the innominate rotates posteriorly.

• For a flat PCA, maximum innominate length occurs at 0^0 innominate subluxation, and diminishes as the innominate rotates posteriorly.

In both the AP lumbopelvic and the APFS pelvic projections, the vertical length of the innominate bone increases as it rotates posteriorly about a symphysis pubis axis. The relative increase is greater in the case of the APFS projection, largely because the innominate bone is more off the central ray. This effect would have been more extreme had a bilaterally anteriorly tipped pelvis been depicted, and less apparent - or even reversed - had a bilaterally posteriorly tipped pelvis been illustrated. The degree of innominate torsion also exerts an influence. The numbers above are normalized for a standard 200 mm innominate vertical length. Although a rather massive posterior subluxation is shown for the sake of clarity, the x-ray beam angles are drawn quite accurately for the respective projections.

The data suggest that the conventional wisdom which has the taller innominate on the AP radiograph posteriorly rotated is in need of some refinement. The more bilaterally anteriorly tipped the pelvis, and

PCA	post rotation, degrees	ant rotation, degrees	delta
N	2.2	-2.4	4.6 mm
S	3.3	-3.5	6.8 mm
F	0.9	-1.2	2.1 mm

Table 1. Projected innominate length differences, 2 degrees opposed bilateral innominate subluxation, full-spine radiography.

the more superior the central ray relative to the pelvis, the greater the validity of this dictum. However, the projected vertical length measurement of the posteriorly rotated innominate bone may even decrease in cases where the subject bears a flat PCA, especially using sectional radiography. Full-spine radiography, with an FFD of 72" and the central ray directed toward T6, tends to establish the dictum, whereas sectional lumbopelvic radiography using an FFD of 40" and a central ray directed one inch below the iliac crest tends to refute it. Projected innominate length differentials are minimal for subjects with flat PCAs, or even go against the "rule" when using sectional radiography, in that the posterior innominate may project shorter than its contralateral counterpart. It should also be noted that whether the innominate height changes are negative or positive, in many cases the millimetric values are arguably too small to be considered significant relative to congenital anatomic variation, x-ray positional error, and x-ray marking error.

If one allows the possibility of opposed, bilateral innominate subluxation, with one innominate rotating posterior and the other simultaneously anterior, then both actual and projected left/right innominate vertical length differentials are greater. Table 1 provides a few representative possibilities for subluxation values of 20, anterior and posterior. This is a value probably low enough to lie within the bounds of published anatomical studies on sacroiliac motion. It can be seen that projected innominate length differentials can attain almost 7 mm at the 2^0 subluxation value, assuming a steep PCA and full-spine radiography.

PCA	post rot	ant rot	delta crest	post rot	ant rot	delta PSIS
normal	-2.5	2.3	4.8 mm	-5	4.8	9.8 mm
steep	-1.4	1.2	2.6 mm	-4.3	4.1	8.6 mm
flat	-3.5	3.3	6.8 mm	-5.5	5.4	10.9 mm

Table 2. Actual iliac crest and PSIS differentials, 2 degrees bilateral, opposed rotation of innominates

Although the primary purpose of this study is to calculate projected innominate length changes, tangential data are also generated for the displacement of actual anatomical landmarks as a function of opposed, bilateral innominate subluxation. Table 2 samples a few outcomes, again, at the 2^0 subluxation level. It can be seen that the PSISs displace by a significantly larger amount than the iliac crest peaks, up to 11 mm for subjects with a flat PCA at the 20 subluxation level. The left/right differences that are produced would almost certainly be clinically detectable. It is reassuring that the asymmetry of anatomical landmarks that clinicians report appear to be well within the confines that anatomical studies report for the sacroiliac joints.

Interestingly, although the subjects with steep PCAs show greater innominate length differentials on x-ray, it is the flat PCA subjects who show the greatest asymmetry on physical examination of the iliac crests and PSISs. Radiography only poorly detects intrapelvic torsion in flat PCAs, whereas physical examination is relatively less effective for detecting pelvic torsion in steep PCAs.

It should be noted that these considerations do not provide a rationale for using full-spine as opposed to sectional radiography. The choice between these two protocols involves many other considerations other than the hypothetical utility of x-ray line marking and radiographic positional asymmetry, including but not limited to the occasional need to rule out pathology and visualize congenital variants. Many patients, of course, would be best served by taking no x-rays at all. If, however, an x-ray is to be taken, the full-spine radiograph is the superior projection to show innominate length changes as a function of posterior innominate rotation.

Conclusion

Chiropractors have long claimed that internal disruption of the pelvic bowl is a leading factor in the genesis of more global spinal distortions and patient complaints. Janse and Illi had fashioned sacroiliac joint dysfunction into the cornerstone of their pathomechanical model of human walking. Sacroiliac subluxation remains today an important clinical entity for practitioners of diverse chiropractic techniques. Indeed, a large and growing body of research supports the contention that the sacroiliac joints are capable of intra-articular motion, a point previously found disputable in some quarters. Notwithstanding the importance afforded the sacroiliac subluxation, surprisingly little progress has been made and consensus achieved on the precise pathomechanics and predicted examination findings resulting from it. It is hoped that this study will contribute be of some value in this regard.

NORMAL PELVIC CARRYING ANGLE

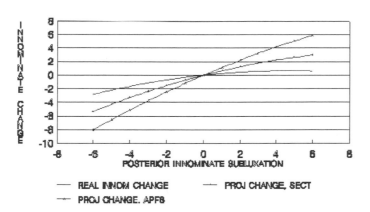

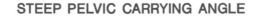

STEEP PELVIC CARRYING ANGLE

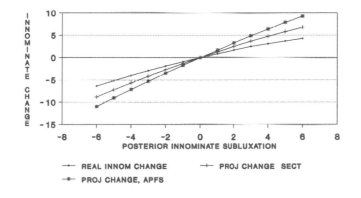

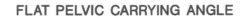

FLAT PELVIC CARRYING ANGLE

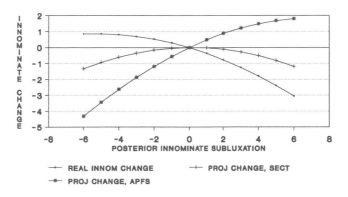

References

1. Herbst, Roger. Gonstead Chiropractic Science & Art. Sci-Chi Publications (publisher unknown, date unknown); p.8

2. Logan, H. B. Textbook of Logan Basic Methods (publisher unknown). Chesterfield. 1951

3. Logan, H. B. Textbook of Logan Basic Methods (publisher unknown). Chesterfield. 1951; p.90

4. Logan, H. B. Textbook of Logan Basic Methods (publisher unknown). Chesterfield. 1951; p.180

5. Herbst, Roger. Gonstead Chiropractic Science & Art. Sci-Chi Publications (publisher unknown, date unknown); p.8

6. Kendall, F.P., McCreary, E.K. Muscles Testing and Function. 3rd ed. Baltimore/London: Williams & Wilkins, 1983; p.291

7. Erhardt, R. Seminar notes (publisher unknown). 1978; p. 183.

8. Hildebrandt, R.W. Chiropractic Spinography. A Manual of Technology and Interpretation. 2nd ed. Williams and Wilkins, Baltimore, 1985; p. 117

9. Jeffery, K.R. X Ray Analysis of Differential Leg Length & Pelvic Distortion. Anglo-European College of Chiropractic dissertation. 1981.

10. Jeffery, K.R. X Ray Analysis of Differential Leg Length & Pelvic Distortion. Anglo-European College of Chiropractic dissertation. 1981; p.23-24

11. Jeffery, K.R. X Ray Analysis of Differential Leg Length & Pelvic Distortion. Anglo-European College of Chiropractic dissertation. 1981; p.23-24

12. Magee, D.J. Orthopedic Physical Assessment. W.B. Saunders Company: Philadelphia, 1987; 306

13. Cibulka, A, Delitto, A, Koldehoff, R. Changes in Innominate Tilt After Manipulation of the Sacroiliac Joint in Patients with Low Back Pain. An Experimental Study. Physical Therapy 1988. 68(9); p.1361

14. Kendall, F.P., McCreary, E.K. Muscles Testing and Function. 3rd ed. Baltimore/London. Williams & Wilkins, 1983; p.275

15. Kapandji, I.A. The Physiology of the Joints. Volume III. The Trunk and Vertebral Column. Churchill Livingstone. New York, 1974: p. 59.

16. Grieve, G. Common Vertebral Joint Problems. Churchill Livingstone. New York. 1981; p.53

17. Jeffery, K.R. X Ray Analysis of Differential Leg Length & Pelvic Distortion. Anglo-European College of Chiropractic dissertation. 1981; p.28

18. Hildebrandt, R.W. Chiropractic Spinography. A Manual of Technology and Interpretation. 2nd ed. Williams and Wilkins, Baltimore, 1985; p.211

19. Herbst, Roger. Gonstead Chiropractic Science & Art. Sci-Chi Publications (publisher unknown, date unknown); p.9

20. Schafer, R.C. Clinical Biomechanics. Musculoskeletal Actions and Reactions. Baltimore/London, Williams and Wilkins, 1987; p. 468

21. Cottingham, J. et al. Shifts in Pelvic Inclination Angle and Parasympathetic Tone Produced by Rolfing Soft Tissue Manipulation. Physical Therapy 1988. 68(9); p.1364 (referring to Ida Rolf's position on the normal innominate carriage).

Appendix 3. Chiropractic listings

In common parlance a "listing" is a direction of tilt, a leaning to one side. Chiropractors have been using this word since the beginning to describe the direction in which a vertebra has misaligned with respect to...with respect to - something! Obviously, a segment can be misaligned only with respect to some other reference point: the segment above or below, the floor, perhaps the central ray of the x-ray tube. It would be an understatement to say that chiropractors have not always been able to agree upon a standard listings system; on the contrary, a rather byzantine discussion over many years has led to very little.

Several factors have interacted to confuse the discussion:

• as mentioned above, there has been a lack of a common reference point for listings;

• there are many different methods for obtaining listings (x-ray, motion palpation, static palpation, muscle palpation, reflex methods employing leg checks, challenges;

• some practitioners use the vertebral body and others use the vertebral spinous process as the reference point for their nomenclatural system.

Nomenclatural Rules or Kinematics?

Certain nomenclatural rules have been adopted merely in order that discussion of mechanical matters may begin. For example, let us suppose that a segment can be seen on a spinograph to reside anteriorward in relationship to the segment below. Should I describe this situation in terms of an anteriority of the superior segment, or a posteriority of the inferior segment? It has become established, among medical doctors as well as chiropractors, that this should be termed an anterolisthesis of the segment above. Unfortunately, this merely nomenclatural rule is seen by many to contain mechanical significance, generally that it is the superior segment which has subluxated, and should be contacted in the event of a corrective thrust.

The terminological convention should not imply that the underlying biomechanical fault resides in the one segment rather than the other, insofar as the subluxation occurs in the joint between the two. Furthermore, there is no a priori reason to suppose that when a clinician attempts to reduce the subluxation by applying a thrust that the force which is applied moves a segment with respect to the one below, any more than with respect to the segment above. Cineradiography has demonstrated that a manipulative thrust introduces a damped disturbance into the spine which extends to several motor units both above and below the point of contact, although it affects the immediately adjacent articulations the most. It's one thing to list L4 with respect to L5, but quite another to suppose that a contact on L4 affects primarily the joint between the two (as opposed to L3-4).

Listing systems

Because of the complexities involved, only the main determinants of a few of the main systems can herein be described. It should be noted that each has various exceptions and "special listings" that embrace specific segments and particular unusual mechanical events. In some ways it turns out that frequently, but certainly not always, discussing listings is tantamount to discussing chiropractic spinography, insofar as many listings are automatically generated by the x-ray line marking analyses peculiar to the given technique. It also turns out that so much of a given technique's mechanical theory - or perhaps lack thereof - is bound up in its listing system, that no critical look may be afforded the latter without simultaneously critiquing the mechanical conceptions themselves. The reader is asked to tolerate the extent to which a mere review of listings devolves into a critical analysis of spinographic technique and mechanical conceptions.

Gonstead

Two points need to be made immediately. First, the Gonstead system posits a certain mechanical assumption (of questionable validity) that underlies everything: a vertebra, in the process of subluxating, first "goes posterior," then possibly "rotates" and finally perhaps "wedges"; this means that all vertebral listings will include a vector of posteriority. Second, the spinous process rather than the body of the vertebra forms the anatomical frame of reference.

Thus, each vertebra (except C1) has a "three letter listing," the first of which is P for posterior, the second of which is either R or L to indicate whether the spinous process has rotated to the left or the right, and the third of which is either S or I to indicate whether the disc plane lines converge or diverge on the side of spinous rotation. For instance, the typical listing "PRS L2" signifies that the second lumbar has subluxated posteriorly with respect to L3, and has rotated and laterally flexed its body to the left.

It should be noted that this posteriority need not be observed on the lateral view. Likewise, the possibility of anterior subluxation is more or less dismissed, despite the following facts:

• Vertebra typically glide anterior in forward flexion, and in fact may become fixed in such a state of anterolisthetic flexion;

• Spinographic studies not uncommonly exhibit evidence of spondylolisthesis, both spondylolytic and non-spondylolytic.

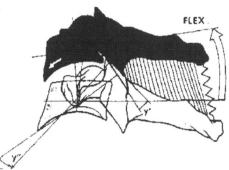

We see in Kapandji's drawing, that forward flexion in the neck is accompanied by anterior glide, creating the possibility of subluxations in which the superior segment is anterior.

In other words, anterior translation is one of the six degrees of freedom available to a vertebral segment; given that a broad consensus of chiropractors would agree that fixation subluxations occur when a segment "freezes" within the range of normal physiological motion, there are a priori reasons to object to the stipulation that posteriority is the rule.

Since the vertebra are constrained to subluxate posteriorly with respect to the segment below, and are barred from subluxating anteriorly, one is at a loss to explain how it is that L5 is permitted to subluxate anteriorly with respect to the sacral base. This lack of parallelism is all the more surprising since the lumbosacral joint is quite homologous to the intervertebral joints in general.

Let us note that the spinous process listings are determined purely in relationship to the central ray of the x-ray tube, so that a given segment that is not rotated with respect to the segment above or below will nonetheless be assigned a rotational malposition listing merely because it happens to be laterally tipped "off the level base." In other words, once it has been determined that a segment must indeed be listed - whether because the spinograph shows it has "wedged," or perhaps because there are clinical findings (instrumentation, palpation, etc.), its rotation is assessed by noting the location of the spinous process relative to the pedicles and the width of the vertebra considered in isolation from adjacent vertebrae.

The innominate bones are listed first as having gone either posteroinferior or anterosuperior, and then "internal" or "external" (medial or lateral) at the sacroiliac joint. The anatomical unlikelihood of a posteriorinferolateral subluxation or an anterosuperomedial subluxation is not considered, in spite of the fact that the sacroiliac joints converge posteriorly rather than align parallel to the sagittal plane.

The sacrum is listed with respect to the sacroiliac articulations or the lumbosacral joint. In the case of the "posterior sacrum," there is no mutual opposed innominate rotation, but the sacrum is said to have rotated posteriorly in the plane of its base on one side: in a P-L sacrum, the sacral base is posterior on the left, and the sacral tubercles are rotated to the right. After having rotated posteriorly, the sacral base may subluxate inferiorly as well, giving rise to the listing PI-L, meaning the sacrum is posterior and inferior on the left. No consideration is given to the possibility of an anterior sacrum (as described by Logan), and no consideration is given to the anatomical limitation that the sacral base, which is wider anteriorly than posteriorly, would force the ilia apart by a wedge action were it to subluxate posteriorly, an occurrence that would be strongly opposed by the powerful sacroiliac ligament.

The sacral listing with respect to the fifth lumbar vertebra is a "posterior sacral base," or "base posterior." Herbst (Sacral Misalignments, p.46) distinguishes a posterior sacral base from a spondylolytic spondylolisthesis of L5 in language that suggests that the Gonstead base posterior is in fact a nonspondylolytic spondylolisthesis. No consideration is given to the possibility of an anteriority of the sacral base with respect to the innominate bone.

The atlas listings are essentially identical to the listing system developed by toggle practitioners, and is described below in the section devoted to them. However, an important distinction in the interpretation of the listing needs to be made: the Gonstead listing is of atlas with respect to axis, whereas the upper cervical practitioners are listing atlas with respect to the occiput. Herbst writes: "A prevalent belief among many chiropractors is that when the atlas becomes subluxated it does so by slipping out from under, and thereby misaligning with, the occiput... [whereas in reality] an atlas subluxation occurs from the atlas misaligning with the axis." The occiput, more or less like a vertebra, is said to wedge and rotate with respect to atlas, after having flexed anteriorly or extended.

Before leaving this description of Gonstead listings, we should mention that it is in very common use, not only among Gonstead clinicians but among Diversified and many other practitioners as well. As has been briefly mentioned above, certain anatomic, referential, and terminological ambiguities and uncertainties exist within it that wind up contradicting important tenets of other listing systems, including that of Logan and of Thompson. In the next unit we offer up a reconciliatory model, one which departs from certain conventional belief systems concerning the interpretation of the various listing systems, but which more than makes up for the departure by uniting them mechanically.

Toggle/Upper Cervical

Atlas listings are derived from an analytic x-ray series: an upper cervical specific series, consisting of a lateral cervical, a vertex, and a nasium view. The nasium view is taken with caudad tube tilt, at an angle conforming to the plane line of atlas that is visualized in the lateral view. The vertex view is taken with the central ray more or less perpendicular to the surface of atlas.

Atlas listings consist of four letters. The first letter is always A, to indicate that when atlas subluxates it always glides anterior with respect to the occipital condyles. The second letter is either S or I, depending on whether the lateral view atlas plane line has tilted superior or inferior with respect to some norm (what norm?). The third letter is either L or R, depending on whether the nasium view shows the atlas to have translated either right or left with respect to the occipital condyles. The fourth and final letter is either P or A, denoting whether the atlas transverse process has rotated anteriorly or posteriorly on the side of laterality, as seen on the vertex view; this information is derived either from a vertex view or from the nasium, where it may be deduced based on the relative widths of the lateral masses (the wider lateral mass is said to be anterior).

Logan Technique

In the end the Logan practitioner is going to list and quantify the degree of sacral inferiority, taking into account other mechanical complications such as "true pelvic anteriority." Neo-Logan practitioners, like Gonstead, have developed a full spine method of analyzing spinographs. Given that Logan mechanotherapeutics are almost entirely devoted to normalizing the inferiority of the sacrum (using the "Basic Contact" on the sacral apex and possibly a heel or sole lift to normalize the inferior sacrum) not surprisingly the spinographic analysis and the listings that are generated by it greatly emphasize the lumbopelvic area. The x-ray marking system is considerably more subtle than the Gonstead system which developed out of it, in that Logan has internal rules for detecting and "correcting" x-ray distortional effects that arise from the subject being off-center with respect to the central ray of the x-ray tube. Gonstead has borrowed correctional rules for pelvic torsional effects on femur head height (whether these rules are right or wrong) but not for left/right off centering.

In terms of listings, we need only mention that the determination of vertebral rotation depends on the location of the spinous process not with respect to the central ray, as in Gonstead, but with respect to the location of the spinous processes above and below. Barge uses the same system throughout the spine, measuring the distance between the lateral aspect of the vertebra and the spinous process, comparing the left/right measurements for analogous measurements above and below. (See any of Dr. Barge's three related books, *Torticollis, Tortipelvis* or Scoliosis.)

Diversified

There isn t really a definite constituted Diversified listings system, anymore than there is a clearly defined Diversified technique per se. More often than not these practitioners employ Gonstead listings, using the spinous processes as reference points, with the main exception occurring in the neck where malpositions are designated with respect to the vertebral bodies. The vertebra are listed as "body right" or "body left" with respect to the segment below. A typical listing might be 'RPI" - body posterior on the right, closed wedge. As compared with Gonstead listings less information is conveyed, insofar as no information is presented concerning lateral curvatures ("wedging") should there be any present. The Gonstead doctor employs a line of drive that is toward the convexity of the spine, using a segmental contact point that takes the rotatory component into account, whereas the Diversified doctor simply adjusts (at least in the neck) according to the direction of vertebral rotation, not taking wedging into account. (We will explore the mechanical consequences of this methodology in the unit concerned with the cervical spine.)

Diversified practitioners, in addition to borrowing Gonstead listings, quite commonly make use of Derifield listings that are often imported from the context of the Thompson technique. (These latter will be examined below, in the unit devoted to the Derifield leg check and Thompsonian derivations.) There is a certain logic to this, insofar as Thompson and allied drop-table practitioners are phylogenetically within the Diversified camp. The use of the table does not itself alter the fundamental chiropractic world view of the practitioners: segments misalign, possibly resulting in nerve interference; the doctor adjusts the segment back toward "correction." Little if any attention is devoted to posture, and even less to the pathophysiology of the subluxation or kinetics of the correction (apart from the empty vague assertion that 'the table does the work." In other words, there is no constituted Diversified theory in the same sense for instance that there is a Logan, Gonstead, or Biomechanics theory.

Thompson Technique

Pelvic syndrome is said to exist when the physiological short leg seems to lengthen with respect to the other when the patient s legs are flexed to approximately 90 degrees in the prone position. Cervical syndrome is said to exist when turning the prone patient s head to either the right or the left changes the apparent length of the legs. The syndrome is named according to which direction of rotation evens the apparent leg length, so that "right cervical syndrome" exists when turning the head to the right evens a short right or left leg. The doctor will locate a "painful nodule (or "taut and tender fibers") on the exposed side of the neck. The doctor s adjustment is applied to the lamina of the involved vertebra, which is to say he adjusts the segment as a "body left/right" according to the Diversified system of nomenclature.

It has occasionally been suggested that whereas pelvic positive would signify a "PI" ilium, pelvic negative would signify an "AS" ilium. Thompson himself appears to believe the latter to denote some sort of PI ilium with "sacral involvement," or some entity involving primarily hamstring spasm. It is our opinion (developed in the unit concerned with the Derifield leg check and Thompsonism) that both pelvic negative and pelvic positive signify PI iliums of possibly different ilk - but are still both PI iliurns. We have a vested interest, now that we have greatly complicated the mechanical model of the PT ilium PDS, to cling to a few empirical "rules," where it appears that the old and new conceptions coincide. It would be nice if we could agree that a physiological short leg, *ceterus paribus*, almost always indicates a PI ilium.

Pierce-Stillwagon technique very much resembles the Thompson work. It adds to the Thompson listings repertoire the "Double AS" and "Double PI" listings. which should not be understood as double sacroiliac lesions, but rather as lumbopelvic. x-ray derived descriptions of the overall arrangement. Double AS patients are hyperlordotic in the lumbar spine, whereas Double P1 patients are hypolordotic. Pierce adds the C5 listing, and thus the C5 adjustment, to the blend. At the end of the chapter is a flow chart showing how a typical drop table practice processes its patients, mostly drawn from a Pierce-Stillwagon technique manual. The reader is also referred to my article on the Thompson Technique, published in the journal *Chiropractic Technique.*

Motion Palpation

Several systems have been developed that have in common the fact that it is the function of the motor unit, rather than the position of any particular bone, that forms the reference point for the listing. A segment is listed as hypomobile or hypermobile with respect to the segment below, in one or more of the available motions that are theoretically possible. There are three possibilities for linear translation and three axes around which rotation make take place.

It should be noted that the practitioners of this type of listings system tend not to be overly concerned with the static initial spatial relationships that typify a given motor unit when they evaluate motion. In other words, a given articulation may exhibit hyperextension (by some definition) in the "neutral" position, but what concerns the examiner is whether starting from this position a segment is able to flex and extend normally. A hyperextended motor unit which nonetheless can be assessed to maintain normal dynamic extensibility would be found normal in that regard, and it might turn out to be hypomobile in forward flexion (for example).

Houston Codes

This system of listings was originally developed by Howe and Hildebrandt to describe for the most part spinographic findings, although some of the categories refer to motor units that display aberrant motion. Although seemingly straight-forward, this listings system has been poorly received by many chiropractors who see it as somehow "pro-medical." (Representative quotation: "At this date 11970s1 the Americans who had this method forced on them by Medicare, are finding it very hard to live with due to the previously mentioned difficulty in constantly proving the subluxation. May we in Canada never fall into this trap. The listings in themselves are essentially self-explanatory and are as follows:

A. Static intersegmental subluxations
    1. Flexion malposition
    2. Extension malposition
    3. Lateral flexion malposition
    4. Rotational malposition
    5. Anterolisthesis
    6. Retrolisthesis
    7. Lateralisthesis
    8. Altered interosseous spacing (decreased/increased)
    9. Osseous foraminal encroachments

B. Kinetic intersegmental subluxations
    I. Hypomobility (fixation subluxation)
    2. Hypermobility (loosened vertebral motor unit)
    3. Aberrant motion

C. Sectional subluxation
    1. Scoliosis and/or alterations of curves secondary to muscular imbalance
    2. Scoliosis and/or alterations of curves secondary to structural asymmetries
    3. Decompensation of adaptational curvatures
    4. Abnormalities of motion

D. Paravertebral subluxations
  1. Costovertebral and costotransverse disrelationships
  2. Sacroiliac subluxations

Right-handed Orthagonal (Cartesian) System

This system was proposed by White and Panjabi. Chiropractors have by and large have found it too cumbersome to use, although Don Harrison (Biophysics technique) has endorsed it and the ACA Council on Technique has expressed serious interest in it. The typical clinician seems to feel that however useful this system is from a mathematical or biomechanical point of view, it does not improve upon traditional listing languages in a way that benefits field practitioners.

It is agreed as a convention that the coordinate system for describing the kinematics of the human spine is structured as follows: the origin is between the cornua of the sacrum. The x axis is horizontal and runs left/right, and is the axis about which forward flexion and extension takes place; the y axis is vertical and is the axis about which axial twisting takes place; and the z axis is, which is also horizontal, projects forward and back, and is the axis about which lateral bending takes place. The sagittal plane is determined by the z-y axes, the frontal plane by the x-y axes, and the transverse plane by the z-x axes. Movements that are forward along z, to the left along x, and up along y are defined as positive linear translations, and opposite directions of motion are defined as negative in value. Likewise, clockwise rotations about an axis are defined as + or - theta (theta is the angle of rotation), with the observer assumed to be standing at the origin looking in the direction of the positive direction of the axis. For example, + theta x corresponds to forward flexion, and right lateral flexion is + theta z.

Coupling is said to occur when a vertebra exhibits motion in more than one degree of freedom simultaneously, as when the cervical vertebrae translate anteriorly during flexion of the neck, forward (+ theta x coupled with +z). The fact that coupling occurs implies that the axis of rotation which may be described for a particular vertebral motion may itself be a function of time, in that its precise location changes during the time interval in which motion occurs.

Sacro-Occipital Technique

SOT is a vast technique, with lots of nooks and crannies. We do not dare get involved with nomenclature in the limited time and space available here, but we should mention the "category" system of patient classification. For a fuller description, with citations, see my article on SOT, published in the journal

Chiropractic Technique.

The category system serves as the lynch-pin of structural correction, while Chiropractic Manipulative Reflex Technique (CMRT) represents the mainstay of somatovisceral intervention. From a diagnostic point of view, the ascription of patients to one of three possible "categories" is central. Category I, "the first level of subluxation to develop" would involve failed coordination between the "sacroiliac respiratory motion" and the "cranial sacral respiratory mechanism," which are normally connected by virtue of the dural membranes and the flow of cerebral spinal fluid. Category II, following on the heels of an unresolved Category I subluxation, involves the "weight-bearing" function of the sacroiliac joint, and is essentially a post-traumatic clinical entity. It would "affect the connective tissue of the cranial sutures and spine, the iliofemoral ligaments, the extremities, and the psoas muscle." An unresolved Category II may progress to a Category III, characterized as an insult to the lumbosacral cartilaginous system, accompanied by nerve root compression or stretch syndrome, injury to "disc tissue, the surrounding muscles, the sciatic nerve and the pyriformis muscles."

Instantaneous axis of rotation

The term instantaneous axis of rotation (IAR) has been defined to embrace this concept: this axis is perpendicular to the plane in which the rigid body moves. The perpendicular bisectors of any two lines connecting the original and new positions of any two points in the body determine this axis (again, see White and Panjabi). The location of this line and the angle describes the motion.

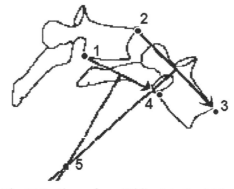

The IAR. Figure from White AA, Panjabi MM. Clinical Biomechanics of the Spine. 1st ed. Philadelphia PA: J. B. Lippincott Company; 1978.White and Pandjabi

18090697R00137

Made in the USA
Charleston, SC
15 March 2013